THE LANGUAGE OF YOGA

The Language of Yoga

Complete A to Y Guide to Āsana Names, Sanskrit Terms, and Chants

Nicolai Bachman

SOUNDS TRUE

Sounds True, Inc.
Boulder CO 80306

Sounds True is a registered trademark of Sounds True, Inc.

This is one of a series of Sanskrit pronunciation guides
by Nicolai Bachman/Sanskrit Sounds.

The purpose of this project is to preserve and encourage the correct spelling and pronunciation of Sanskrit terms related to the science of yoga.

For information about classes, workshops, or other products, please contact Sanskrit Sounds, Santa Fe, New Mexico, www.SanskritSounds.com

Sanskrit translations by Nicolai Bachman.

Digitally recorded, edited, and mastered at Santa Fe Soundworks.

Printed in Korea

ISBN: 1-59179-281-9

Originally published as *Āsana Names and the Language of Yoga,* © Nicolai Bachman, Sanskrit Sounds, Santa Fe, New Mexico, 2004

Bachman, Nicolai.
The language of yoga: complete A–Y guide to āsana names, sanskrit terms, and chants / Nicolai Bachman.
Includes index.
ISBN 1-59179-281-9
Library of Congress Control Number: 2005928672

Thank You

David Frawley
Tias and Sūrya Little
Jeff Martens
Tim Miller
Darlene Tate

and especially
my wife, Margo,
for her ever-present support and love.

TABLE OF CONTENTS

	TRACK	PAGE
Introduction		1
DISC 1: THE LANGUAGE OF YOGA		
Chants for Your Practice		7
Gaṇānāṃ Tvā	1	9
Chant to Sarasvatī	2	10
Yogena Cittasya	3	11
Vande Gurūṇām	4	12
Maṅgala Mantra	5	13
Śiva Mantra	6	14
Chant to Kṛṣṇamācārya	7	15
Yoga Sūtras of Patañjali	8	16
Yoga Terms		17
Aṣṭāṅga	9	18
Yamas	10	19
Niyamas	11	19
Animals	12	20
Bandhas	13	21
Body Parts	14	22
Cakras	15	23
Deities and Sages	16	24
Directions and Positions	17	25
Dṛṣṭis	18	26
Elements	19	27
Kleśas	20	27
Mudrās	21	28
Numbers	22	30
Prāṇāyāma	23	31
Ṣaṭ-Karmas	24	32

TABLE OF CONTENTS

	TRACK	PAGE
Texts	25	33
Upaniṣads	26	34
Vāyus	27	35
Vedas	28	35
General Yoga Terms	29	36

DISC 2: ĀSANA NAMES

	TRACK	PAGE
Aṣṭāṅga Sequences		43
Aṣṭāṅga First Series		45
Invocation Chant: Vande Gurūṇām	1	45
Sun-Salutation A	2	46
Sun-Salutation B	3	47
Standing Postures	4	48
Seated Postures	5	50
Finishing Postures	6	53
Aṣṭāṅga First Series Summary		55
Aṣṭāṅga Second Series	7	56
Aṣṭāṅga Second Series Summary		60
Aṣṭāṅga Third Series	8	61
Aṣṭāṅga Third Series Summary		65

Āsana Names 67

	TRACK	PAGE
A	9	69
B	10	72
C	11	75
D	12	77
E	13	79
G	14	82
H	15	84
J	16	85
K	17	86
L	18	89
M	19	90
N	20	92
P	21	93
R	22	100
S	23	101
T	24	107
U	25	109
V	26	113
Y	27	116

TABLE OF CONTENTS

	TRACK	PAGE
Indices		117
Āsana Name Synonyms	28	118
English Name Index		120
Sanskrit Alphabet	29	138

INTRODUCTION

Knowing how to properly pronounce Sanskrit is a crucial skill for serious students and teachers of yoga.

This sacred language originated from oral traditions developed to communicate the spiritual insights of ancient sages. Because Sanskrit is the language of yoga, understanding key Sanskrit terminology and its pronunciation can deepen a practitioner's knowledge of the yogic path. It can also provide a more complete understanding of the meaning and purpose of yoga *āsanas*, or postures—an understanding that is lost when these āsanas are known only by their English names.

Sanskrit is said to have been divinely revealed to meditating sages thousands of years ago. One story tells of Śiva beating his *damaru* drum fourteen times and creating the Sanskrit alphabet. These fourteen "Maheśvara Sūtras" form the beginning of the text defining Sanskrit grammar. The alphabet is perfectly designed for the human vocal apparatus, and the sound of each word represents the subtle energy of its meaning. Because each syllable is either one or two beats, pronouncing correctly allows one to feel the natural rhythm of the language and imbibe the true essence of the word. Sanskrit is called *Devavāṇi* or "language of the Gods" because it is said that the Gods understand and communicate in Sanskrit. Thus, sacred ceremonies like births, weddings, deaths, and religious rituals all involve Sanskrit chanting. The sound of the Vedic hymns is their life, preserved by thousands of generations through chanting.

Because Vedic wisdom was passed down orally long before it was written, no one knows when it actually began. The Vedas are the earliest known Sanskrit writings, beginning with the Ṛg Veda whose written form dates back to at least 1500 BCE. The subsequent three Vedas (Sāma, Yajur, and Atharva) are all derived from the Ṛg Veda. The Upaniṣads, which form the basis for Vedānta philosophy, are extrapolations and summaries of the Vedas. Taken together, the Vedas and their offspring Upaniṣads are known as *sruti,* meaning "heard," because they are considered to be of divine origin, originally revealed by enlightened seers.

Yoga, along with *Āyurveda* (Indian medicine), *Jyotiṣa* (Indian astrology), and countless other branches of Vedic wisdom, was passed down orally and literally using the refined Sanskrit language. *Sūtras,* terse aphorisms packed with information and easy to memorize, were often composed to record ideas in the most efficient way possible. Only with the help of a teacher and/or a commentary could a student learn the depth of their meaning. Verses were also written in rhythmic meters, most commonly four lines of either eight or eleven syllables each. Chanting or singing these verses provides another natural and easy way to remember them by heart.

Yoga in the West is often largely focused on practicing physical postures (āsanas). However, āsana is in fact only one of eight distinct limbs of yoga (see Aṣṭāṅga). Knowing the posture names in Sanskrit allows teachers and students to unambiguously refer to a posture. Using the English translation as the reference may be confusing because translations can differ—the same posture may have several different English names. In addition, fully comprehending all parts of an āsana name can provide a deeper understanding of its form and function. Noticing how the same word is used in several different posture names will reveal subtle nuances that would otherwise be lost. The Indian process of learning is largely based on viewing an object from a variety of angles, thus seeing it in its complete form.

The purpose of this book is to preserve and encourage the correct sound and spelling of Sanskrit chants and terms related to the science of yoga. This provides a reference for yoga practitioners who wish to perpetuate the vocabulary of yoga in an accurate and respectful way. Seeing terms grouped together in logical arrangements allows one to visualize their relationship to each other.

We hope your journey on the path of yoga will expand and brighten as you experience the audio and visual energy of this beautiful language.

SANSKRIT PRONUNCIATION NOTES

Vowel combining: In Sanskrit, when two vowels meet they will combine into something else. For example, "paścima uttānāsana" becomes "paścimottānāsana" and "marīci āsana" becomes "marīcyāsana."

Consonant combining: In Sanskrit, if the final consonant of one word is not sound-compatible with the initial consonant of the next word, the final consonant may change. For example, "ṣaṭ mukhī" becomes "ṣanmukhī," "tiryac mukha" becomes "tiryaṅmukha," and "catur pāda" becomes "catuṣpāda."

Some Sanskrit sounds are pronounced slightly differently in North and South India. The "v" might sound like a "w" and the "ś" or "ṣ" may sound like a "sh" or a "s."

There are some differences between Sanskrit and Hindi pronunciation. In Sanskrit, when a word ends with an "a," the "a" is pronounced. In Hindi it is often dropped, even though it is written the same way. For example, the Sanskrit "āsana" sounds like "āsan" in Hindi.

SANSKRIT	HINDI
"a" at the end of a word is pronounced	"a" at the end of a word is often not pronounced
"ā" at the end of a word is long	"ā" at the end of a word is pronounced a short "a"
"ph" pronounced as an aspirated "p"	"ph" pronounced like "f"

EXPLANATORY NOTES

The images at the beginning of each section are the geometrical representations (*yantra*) of each elemental *cakra*. Each yantra conveys the energy that matches the associated cakra. The Sanskrit sound in the center of each yantra is that cakra's primary sound, a single syllable ending in "m."

SECTION	CAKRA LOCATION	ELEMENT	PRIMARY SANSKRIT SOUND
Chants for Your Practice	throat	space	haṃ
Yoga Terms	heart	air	yaṃ
Aṣṭāṅga Sequences	navel	fire	raṃ
Āsana Names	reproductive area	water	vaṃ
Indices	base of the spine	earth	laṃ

If you cannot find the Sanskrit āsana name in the A–Y section, look in the Āsana Name Synonyms index (page 118). Use the English Name Index on page 120 to locate the posture by English name.

The line drawings are intended as a general representation of each posture. Some variations are not shown. Many postures have several different names, and one name may be used for many postures. The names included here are drawn from the classical systems of yoga and the teachings of B.K.S. Iyengar and T.K.V. Desikachar. The first three series of K. Pattabhi Jois' Aṣṭāṅga system are given separately.

Many Sanskrit terms are very complex and difficult to translate into English. Because of this, the suggested meanings are not meant to be definitive. I chose to provide the literal definition for most āsana names. For yoga terms whose common meaning is different than the literal, the literal meaning is shown in quotation marks.

AṢṬĀṄGA SEQUENCES

In Sanskrit the consonants are used to count variations of a posture. So ka=a, kha=b, ga=c, gha=d.

Several postures are not specifically named in the series but are done as transitory postures.These are indicated with an asterisk*.

Many teachers have modified the first series in different ways, usually adding or deleting postures. The first series presented here is based on K. Pattabhi Jois' own writing in Sanskrit. The second and third series are consistent and drawn from the knowledge of senior practitioners.

The first and last postures (Samasthiti and Utpluti) are pronounced with an "h" on the end by most practitioners. Even though this is inconsistent with the remaining āsana names (which are not pronounced with their ending "m"), out of respect for convention it remains that way here.

Many names in the third series are different than in the A–Y section. For example, "paścimottānāsana" in the A–Y section is spelled "paścimatānāsana" in the Aṣṭāṅga section.

CHANTS FOR YOUR PRACTICE

Seven common chants
recited as part
of a yoga class

Seven yoga sūtras
relating to the
definition of
yoga and āsana

Sanskrit is a very rhythmic and musical language that lends itself well to singing and chanting. Each syllable is either short (one beat) or long (two beats). Recording the ancient wisdom in standard meters enabled easy memorization via chanting, and therefore provided a useful means of preserving Vedic wisdom over time. The first chant, to Gaṇeśa, is from the Ṛg Veda, the oldest Sanskrit text, written over 3500 years ago. You can tell that it is a Vedic chant by the tonal marks above and below the letters. A horizontal line below a syllable indicates a low tone, no mark means a middle tone, and a vertical line above denotes a high tone. If there are two vertical lines above, you use a middle tone for the first beat, then a high tone for the second beat. Follow the written text as you listen to the CD and you will hear the three tones clearly.

The vast majority of Sanskrit verses are written in meter, usually four lines long with each line being a set number of syllables. The most common meters have either eight or eleven syllables in each line. All chants included here except the first two are in eight or eleven syllable meter.

The sound *Oṁ* is thought to be the original sound from which the entire manifest universe began. Om itself is believed to contain all other sounds and therefore all forms of energy. It is very common to begin and end a chant with Om.

Chanting to a deity invokes that deity's energy, and is an auspicious way to begin a practice or endeavor. Traditionally, throughout India, Gaṇeśa is worshipped first, being the remover of obstacles and bestower of goodness and abundance. After a chant to Gaṇeśa, one performs a chant appropriate to a particular activity, whether it be a practice, meditation, new undertaking, etc. All chants should be recited with a respectful and devotional attitude.

Gaṇānāṃ Tvā (Ṛgveda 2.23.1)

A mantra to Gaṇeśa, the elephant-headed deity who removes obstacles and grants protection.

DISC 1, TRACK 1

ॐ	Om
गणानां त्वा गणपतिं हवामहे	gaṇānāṃ tvā gaṇapatiṃ havāmahe,
कविं कवीनामुपमश्रवस्तमम् ।	kaviṃ kavīnām upamaśravastamaṃ,
ज्येष्ठराजं ब्रह्मणां ब्रह्मणस्पत	jyeṣṭha-rājaṃ brahmaṇāṃ brahmaṇaspata
आ नः शृण्वन्नूतिभिस्सीद सादनम् ॥	ā naḥ śṛṇvannūtibhissīda sādanam.
श्रीमहागणपतये नमः	śrī-mahā-gaṇapataye namaḥ

Among all of Śiva's attendants, we invoke you Gaṇeśa,
the seer of seers, the most glorious and eminent,
sovereign of all brahmans. Oh Lord of Brahman,
having heard us, sit nearby with all (your) protective energies.
Salutations to the great and magnificent Gaṇeśa!

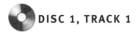

Chant to Sarasvatī

To invoke the energy of speech and learning.

DISC 1, TRACK 2

या कुन्देन्दुतुषारहारधवला	yā kundendu-tuṣārahāra-dhavalā
या शुभ्रवस्त्रावृता ।	yā śubhra-vastrāvṛtā,
या वीणावरदण्डमण्डितकरा	yā vīṇāvara-daṇḍa-maṇḍita-karā
या श्वेतपद्मासना ॥	yā śveta-padmāsanā.
या ब्रह्माच्युतशङ्करप्रभृतिभिर्	yā brahmācyutaśaṅkara-prabhṛtibhir
देवैः सदा वन्दिता ।	devaiḥ sadā vanditā,
सा मां पातु सरस्वती भगवती	sā māṃ pātu Sarasvatī bhagavatī
निश्शेषजाड्यापहा ॥	niśśeṣajāḍyāpahā.

Who is pure white like a garland of jasmine, the moon or snow,
covered with white clothing;
whose hands are decorated with a vīṇā, boon, and staff,
seated on a white lotus;
ever worshipped by the gods led by Brahma, Viṣṇu, and Śiva;
may she, divine Sarasvatī, who removes all darkness, protect me.

Yogena Cittasya

To Patañjali, author of the *Yoga Sūtras*. Often chanted at the beginning of a yoga practice or sūtra class.

DISC 1, TRACK 3

योगेन चित्तस्य पदेन वाचां	yogena cittasya padena vācāṃ
मलं शरीरस्य च वैद्यकेन ।	malaṃ śarīrasya ca vaidyakena,
यो ऽपाकरोत्तं प्रवरं मुनीनां	yo 'pākarottaṃ pravaraṃ munīnāṃ
पतञ्जलिं प्राञ्जलिरानतो ऽस्मि ॥	Patañjaliṃ prāñjalirānato 'smi.
आबाहुपुरुषाकारं	ābāhu puruṣākāraṃ
शङ्खचक्रासिधारिणम् ।	śaṅkha-cakrāsi-dhāriṇaṃ,
सहस्रशिरसं श्वेतं	sahasra-śirasaṃ śvetaṃ
प्रणमामि पतञ्जलिम् ॥	praṇamāmi Patañjalim.
श्रीमते अनन्ताय नागराजाय नमो नमः	Śrīmate anantāya nāgarājāya namo namaḥ

I am a deep bow with hands folded to Patañjali,
the most excellent of sages, who removed
impurity of consciousness through yoga,
impurity of speech through word (grammar), and
impurity of the body through medicine (Āyurveda).

In the form of a man up to the shoulders,
holding the conch (divine sound), discus (wheel of time),
and sword (discrimination),
thousand-headed, white,
I bow respectfully to Patañjali.

To the magnificent endless one, the king of the nāgas,
salutations, salutations.

Vande Gurūṇām

Devotion to the lotus feet of all gurus, equated with Śiva. Second half to Patañjali, considered an incarnation of Viṣṇu. Often chanted at the beginning of a yoga practice.

DISC 1, TRACK 4

वन्दे गुरूणां चरणारविन्दे	vande gurūṇāṃ caraṇāravinde
संदर्शितस्वात्मसुखावबोधे ।	saṃdarśita-svātma-sukhāvabodhe,
निःश्रेयसे जाङ्गलिकायमाने	niḥśreyase jāṅgalikāyamāne
संसारहालाहलमोहशान्त्यै ॥	saṃsāra-hālāhala-moha-śāntyai.
आबाहुपुरुषाकारं	ābāhu puruṣākāraṃ
शङ्खचक्रासिधारिणम् ।	śaṅkha-cakrāsi-dhāriṇaṃ,
सहस्रशिरसं श्वेतं	sahasra-śirasaṃ śvetaṃ
प्रणमामि पतञ्जलिम् ॥	praṇamāmi Patañjalim.

I worship the lotus feet of all the gurus,
which awaken and manifest joy in oneself;
beyond comparison, appearing as a snake-charmer (Śiva)
for pacifying the poisonous delusion of saṃsāra (the cycle of birth and death).

In the form of a man up to the shoulders,
holding the conch (divine sound), discus (wheel of time),
and sword (discrimination),
thousand-headed, white,
I bow respectfully to Patañjali.

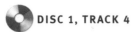

Maṅgala Mantra (Auspicious Mantra)

Often chanted at the end of a yoga practice.

DISC 1, TRACK 5

स्वस्ति प्रजाभ्यः परिपालयन्तां
न्यायेन मार्गेण महीं महीशाः ।
गोब्राह्मणेभ्यः शुभमस्तु नित्यं
लोकाः समस्ताः सुखिनो भवन्तु ॥

svasti prajābhyaḥ paripālayantāṃ
nyāyena mārgeṇa mahīṃ mahīśāḥ,
gobrāhmaṇebhyaḥ śubhamastu nityaṃ
lokāḥ samastāḥ sukhino bhavantu.

Hail to the creators!
May (these) great lords protect the earth properly and justly.
May one be eternally fortunate due to cows (wealth) and Brahmans.
May all worlds be happy.

Śiva Mantra (from Nirālamba Upaniṣad)

Often chanted at the beginning of a yoga practice.

DISC 1, TRACK 6

ॐ नमः शिवाय गुरवे
सच्चिदानन्दमूर्तये ।
निष्प्रपञ्चाय शान्ताय
निरालम्बाय तेजसे ॥

Om namaḥ Śivāya gurave
saccidānanda-mūrtaye,
niṣprapañcāya śāntāya
nirālambāya tejase.

Salutations to Śiva, the teacher
whose form is truth, consciousness, and bliss,
who is without deceit, tranquil,
independent, and illuminating.

Chant to Kṛṣṇamācārya

Composed by Prof. T. Kṛṣṇamācārya in response to his students' request for a chant that would honor their teacher. Presented here in recognition of Prof. Kṛṣṇamācārya's unparalleled contribution to the understanding and practice of yoga throughout the world.

DISC 1, TRACK 7

श्रीकृष्णवागीशयतीश्वराभ्यां	Śrī-Kṛṣṇa-Vāgīśa-yatīśvarābhyāṃ
संप्राप्तचक्राङ्कनभाष्यसारम् ।	saṃprāpta-cakrāṅkana-bhāṣyasāram,
श्रीनूत्नरङ्गेन्द्रयतौ समर्पितस्वं	Śrī-nūtna-Raṅgendra-yatau samarpitasvaṃ
श्रीकृष्णमार्यं गुरुवर्यमीडे ॥	Śrī-Kṛṣṇam-āryaṃ guruvaryam īḍe.
विरोधे कार्तिके मासे	virodhe kārtike māse
शतताराकृतोदयम् ।	śatatārā-kṛtodayaṃ,
योगाचार्यं कृष्णमार्यं	yogācāryaṃ Kṛṣṇam-āryaṃ
गुरुवर्यमहं भजे ॥	guru-varyam-ahaṃ bhaje.
श्रीगुरुभ्यो नमः	Śrī-gurubhyo namaḥ
हरिः ॐ	Hariḥ Om

I praise (our) principle teacher, the venerable Śrī Kṛṣṇamācārya,
who obtained the essence of Vedānta from Śrī Vāgīśa,
(and) the cakra-marking from Śrī Kṛṣṇa,
both master ascetics (and teachers),
(and) who entrusted himself completely in Śrī Raṅgendra, ascetic (and teacher).

Born in (the year of) Virodha,
during the month of Kārtika
(under the) star of Śata,
to (this) teacher of yoga,
the venerable Śrī T. Kṛṣṇamācārya
(our) principle teacher, I pray.

Yoga Sūtras of Patañjali

Written by Patañjali between 500–200 BCE, this concise set of 196 aphorisms has become the most widely accepted treatise on yoga as a development of human consciousness. Included here are a few sūtras that define yoga and relate to āsana. In the original Sanskrit script, the chapter number and sūtra number are shown at the end of the sūtra and are surrounded by vertical lines called *daṇḍa*. These correspond to the "chapter#.sūtra#" shown below.

DISC 1, TRACK 8

योगश्चित्तवृत्तिनिरोधः ॥ १.२ ॥
1.2 yogaścittavṛttinirodhaḥ
Yoga is stilling the fluctuations in (one's) consciousness.

तदा द्रष्टुः स्वरूपे ऽवस्थानम् ॥ १.३ ॥
1.3 tadā draṣṭuḥ svarūpe 'vasthānam
Then, the abiding of the seer in (its) own true nature.

वृत्तिसारूप्यमितरत्र ॥ १.४ ॥
1.4 vṛttisārūpyamitaratra
Otherwise, conformity/identity with the fluctuations.

यमनियमासनप्राणायामप्रत्याहारधारणाध्यानसमाधयो ऽष्टावङ्गानि ॥ २.२९ ॥
2.29 yamaniyamāsanaprāṇāyāmapratyāhāradhāraṇādhyānasamādhayo `ṣṭāvaṅgāni
The eight limbs are yama, niyama, āsana, prāṇāyāma, pratyāhāra, dhāraṇā, dhyāna, (and) samādhi.

स्थिरसुखमासनम् ॥ २.४६ ॥
2.46 sthirasukhamāsanam
Āsana (has the qualites of) stability and comfort ...

प्रयत्नशैथिल्यानन्तसमापत्तिभ्याम् ॥ २.४७ ॥
2.47 prayatnaśaithilyānantasamāpattibhyām
... due to relaxation with appropriate effort and convergence with the infinite.

ततो द्वन्द्वानभिघातः ॥ २.४८ ॥
2.48 tato dvandvānabhighātaḥ
From that, no disturbance from the pairs of opposites.

YOGA TERMS

A comprehensive list
of Sanskrit words
related to yoga

Each term is repeated twice
with space for you to repeat.

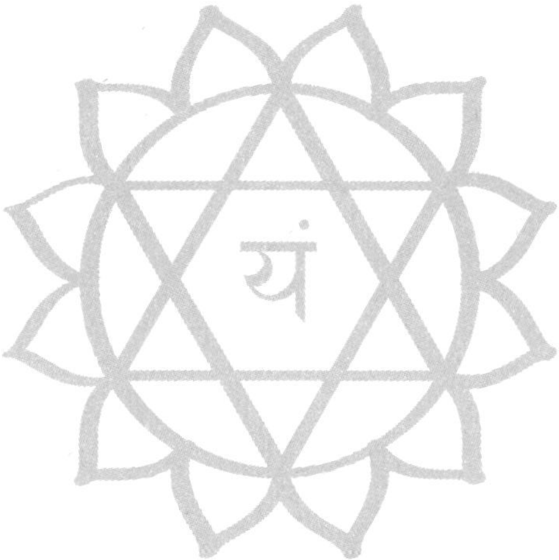

Aṣṭāṅga (eight limbs of yoga)

The term Aṣṭāṅga refers to the eight limbs of yoga, which are described in Patañjali's *Yoga Sūtras.* They provide a practical way of living happily in the world while gradually moving one's consciousness inward. The most external limb comprises the *yamas* (social behaviors). Next are the *niyamas* (personal behaviors), which are like internal yamas. Āsanas (physical postures) keep our body flexible, strong, and healthy. *Prāṇāyāma* (breath regulation) is even more subtle and begins to purify the mind. *Pratyāhāra* (internalization of the senses) brings one further inward by removing sense distractions from the mind. The last three limbs, termed *"antaraṅga,"* meaning "inner limbs," all take place in one's consciousness. *Dhāraṇā* enables one to focus a stream of attention onto a single object. Maintaining this focus for a long time is *dhyāna,* the seventh limb. Finally, when the object of meditation is so completely absorbed in the consciousness that there is no perceived separation between subject and object, *samādhi* is experienced. This is the final goal.

DISC 1, TRACK 9

1	yama	यम	social ethics "restraints" (see Yamas, p. 19)
2	niyama	नियम	personal ethics "internal restraints" (see Niyamas, p. 19)
3	āsana	आसन	posture, sitting
4	prāṇāyāma	प्राणायाम	breath regulation (see Prāṇāyāma section, p. 31)
5	pratyāhāra	प्रत्याहार	internalization of the senses, "drawing back"
6	dhāraṇā	धारणा	focus, concentration
7	dhyāna	ध्यान	maintaining a focus, meditation
8	samādhi	समाधि	complete absorption

Yamas (social ethics)

Yamas are social ethics that allow one to coexist peacefully in community. Nonviolence is the first and foremost ethic.

DISC 1, TRACK 10

ahiṃsā	अहिंसा	nonviolence, reducing harm
satya	सत्य	truth
asteya	अस्तेय	nonstealing
brahmacarya	ब्रह्मचर्य	appropriate use of one's vital energy
aparigraha	अपरिग्रह	nonpossessiveness

Niyamas (personal ethics)

Niyamas are personal ethics necessary for taking care of and developing oneself in order to live a balanced life. Cleanliness and purity of the body, mind, and environment is outermost, followed by an outer and inner contentment. Developing the body through a regular practice, the mind through intellectual stimulation, and the spirit through devotion to a higher power all contribute to personal growth and freedom.

DISC 1, TRACK 11

śauca	शौच	purity, cleanliness
santoṣa	सन्तोष	contentment
tapas	तपस्	practice causing change, "heat"
svādhyāya	स्वाध्याय	self-study/observation (especially mantra)
īśvarapraṇidhāna	ईश्वरप्रणिधान	devotion, surrender to a higher force

Animals

Certain postures are named after the way animals look or are perceived. For example, lion posture looks and feels like a lion roaring loudly with its chest protruding and tongue sticking out.

DISC 1, TRACK 12

baka	बक	crane
bheka	भेक	frog
bhujaṅga	भुजङ्ग	serpent
cakora	चकोर	partridge
garuḍa	गरुड	eagle
go	गो	cow
gorakṣa	गोरक्ष	cowherder, one who tends cows
haṃsa	हंस	swan
kapiñjal̇a	कपिञ्जल	bird that lives on raindrops
kāka	काक	crow
kapota	कपोत	pigeon
kāraṇḍava	कारण्डव	Himalayan goose
krauñca	क्रौञ्च	heron
kukkuṭa	कुक्कुट	rooster
kūrma	कूर्म	tortoise
makara	मकर	sea animal like a crocodile
matsya	मत्स्य	fish
mayūra	मयूर	peacock

nakra	नक्र	crocodile
śalabha	शलभ	locust
śaśa	शश	rabbit
siṃha	सिंह	lion
śvāna	श्वान	dog
tittibha	तित्तिभ	firefly
uṣṭra	उष्ट्र	camel
vātāyana	वातायन	horse
vṛścika	वृश्चिक	scorpion

Bandhas (bindings or locks)

Bandhas are muscular locks created by contracting or squeezing certain muscles, holding them, then releasing them, thereby relaxing that area of the body. Bandhas strengthen and balance the nervous system and subtle body and can be used for a variety of therapeutic effects.

DISC 1, TRACK 13

jālandhara-bandha	जालंधरबन्ध	throat lock "net support"
jihvā-bandha	जिह्वाबन्ध	tongue lock
mūla-bandha	मूलबन्ध	root lock
uḍḍīyāna-bandha	उड्डीयानबन्ध	rising up lock

Body Parts

Many posture names contain the names of body parts. Knowing the individual names of each body part helps one to remember how to do a posture.

DISC 1, TRACK 14

aṅga	अङ्ग	limb
aṅguṣṭha	अङ्गुष्ठ	big toe, thumb
bhuja	भुज	arm
gaṇḍa	गण्ड	cheek, side of face
garbha	गर्भ	womb
hanu	हनु	jaw
hasta	हस्त	hand
jānu	जानु	knee
jaṭhara	जठर	stomach
karṇa	कर्ण	ear
mukha	मुख	face, mouth
pāda	पाद	foot, leg
śīrṣa	शीर्ष	head

Cakras (energy centers)

Cakras are circular vortexes of energy near the spinal cord, transected by the central *suṣumnā nāḍī* through which the *kuṇḍalinī* energy travels upward as consciousness awakens. Each cakra is responsible for a variety of bodily functions and emotions. The cakras listed here are ordered from bottom to top, reflecting the direction of the kuṇḍalinī and the evolution of a yoga practice from gross to subtle.

DISC 1, TRACK 15

1	mūlādhāra	मूलाधार	base of the spine, "root-support"
2	svādhiṣṭhāna	स्वाधिष्ठान	sacrum/reproductive area, "self-established"
3	maṇipūra	मणिपूर	navel area, "filled with jewels"
4	anāhata	अनाहत	heart area, "unstruck"
5	viśuddha	विशुद्ध	throat area, "purified"
6	ājñā	आज्ञा	between the eyebrows; command, will, "enhanced knowledge"
7	sahasrāra	सहस्रार	crown of the head, "one thousand-spoked"

Deities and Sages

Yoga philosophy and Hinduism both have their roots in the Vedas. Many master yoga teachers are Hindu and share stories with their students which metaphorically reveal an idea that the teacher is trying to convey. Thus it is important to know the major characters in the Hindu pantheon.

DISC 1, TRACK 16

Brahman	ब्रह्मन्	energy of creation
Buddha	बुद्ध	awakened one
Durgā	दुर्गा	female aspect of Śiva
Gaṇeśa	गणेश	elephant-headed son of Śiva, scribe of the Mahābhārata, remover of obstacles
Hanumān	हनुमान्	energy of service, monkey-deity servant of Rāma
Kālī	काली	female aspect of Śiva
Patañjali	पतञ्जलि	author of the Yoga Sūtras
Kṛṣṇa	कृष्ण	incarnation of Viṣṇu, main character in Bhagavad-Gītā
Rāma	राम	incarnation of Viṣṇu, main character in the Rāmāyaṇa
Sarasvatī	सरस्वती	energy of speech and learning, wife of Brahma
Śiva	शिव	energy of destruction and transformation
Viṣṇu	विष्णु	energy of preservation and maintenance
Vyāsa	व्यास	author of the Mahābhārata

Directions and Positions

Many posture names contain certain directions and positions. Knowing these helps one to remember how to do a posture.

DISC 1, TRACK 17

adho	अधो	downward
parivartana	परिवर्तन	revolving
parivṛtta	परिवृत्त	revolved
pārśva	पार्श्व	side
paścima	पश्चिम	back, behind, West
prasārita	प्रसारित	spread
pūrva	पूर्व	front, East
sthiti	स्थिति	standing
supta	सुप्त	supine
tiryaṅ	तिर्यङ्	oblique
upaviṣṭa	उपविष्ट	seated
ūrdhva	ऊर्ध्व	upward
utthita	उत्थित	extended
uttāna	उत्तान	out-stretching
viparīta	विपरीत	inverted

Dṛṣṭis (views)

A *dṛṣṭi* is where the gaze is supposed to be focused during a posture. These are more commonly used by Aṣṭāṅga yoga practitioners.

DISC 1, TRACK 18

aṅguṣṭhāgra	अङ्गुष्ठाग्र	tip of the thumb
bhrūmadhya	भ्रूमध्य	between the eyebrows
hastāgra	हस्ताग्र	tip of the hand
nābhicakra	नाभिचक्र	navel cakra
nasāgra	नसाग्र	tip of the nose
pādāgra	पादाग्र	tip of the foot
pārśva	पार्श्व	sideways (far left or far right)
ūrdhva	ऊर्ध्व	upwards

Elements

The "five great elements," called *pañca-mahā-bhūta,* are the basic building blocks of the manifest world. From the most gross element of earth to the most subtle and refined element of space, they represent every possible form of matter.

DISC 1, TRACK 19

pṛthivī	पृथिवी	earth
āp	आप्	water
tejas	तेजस्	fire
vāyu	वायु	air
ākāśa	आकाश	space, ether

Kleśas (afflictions)

In Patanjali's *Yoga Sūtras,* these five afflictions are the cause of future karma and suffering. *Avidyā* (ignorance), the most important, is the field for the others, which can only exist in its presence.

DISC 1, TRACK 20

avidyā	अविद्या	ignorance, "lack of knowledge"
asmitā	अस्मिता	ego, "I am-ness"
rāga	राग	attachment, passion, desire
dveṣa	द्वेष	aversion, dislike
abhiniveśa	अभिनिवेश	will to survive, fear of death

Mudrās (seals or gestures)

Each *mudrā* has a specific energetic. Often fingers touch each other, effectively connecting energy channels (*nāḍīs*) of the body that affect both the gesturer and gesturee.

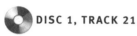

DISC 1, TRACK 21

abhaya-mudrā	अभयमुद्रा	"no fear gesture," palm facing away from you, fingers together	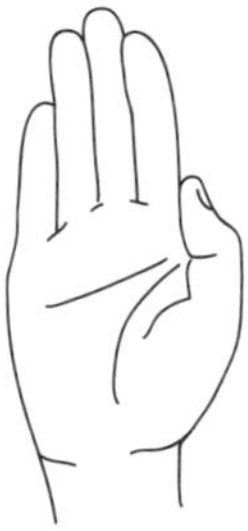
añjali-mudrā	अञ्जलिमुद्रा	"prayer gesture," palms together, fingertips facing upwards	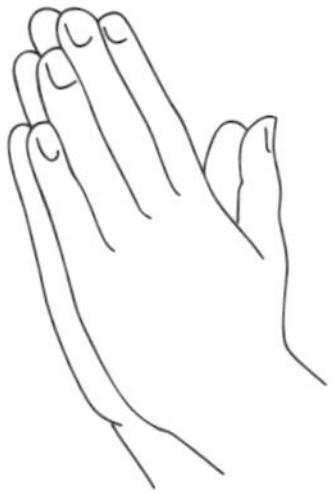
cin-mudrā	चिन्मुद्रा	"consciousness gesture," palms down, index fingertip and thumb-tip touch	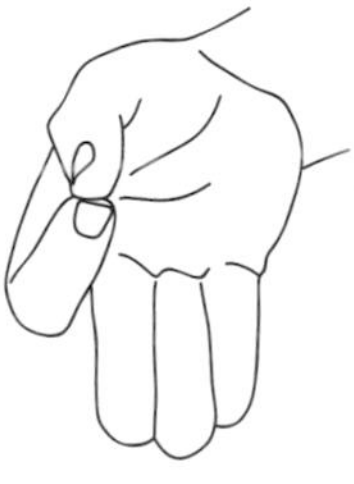
dhyāna-mudrā	ध्यानमुद्रा	"meditation gesture," both palms facing upwards, on the lap, right hand on left, fingers fully stretched	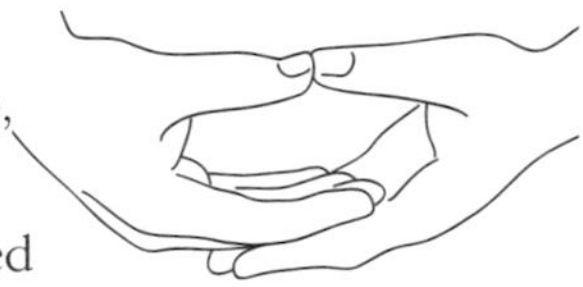

jñāna-mudrā ज्ञानमुद्रा "knowledge gesture," palms up, index fingertip and thumb-tip touch

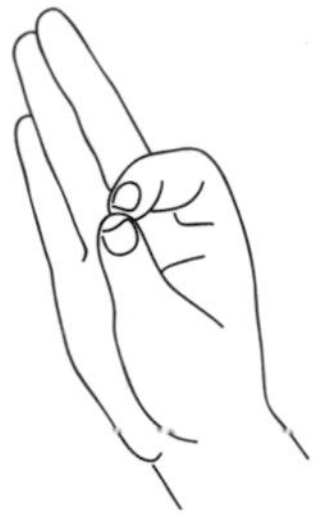

kāraṇa-mudrā कारणमुद्रा "banishing gesture," thumb holds middle two fingers, index and little fingers point out

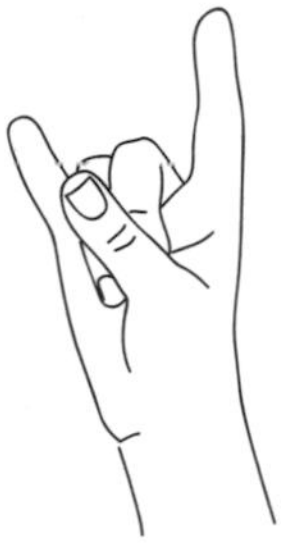

varadā-mudrā वरदामुद्रा "granting a boon gesture," palm faces outward with arm completely extended

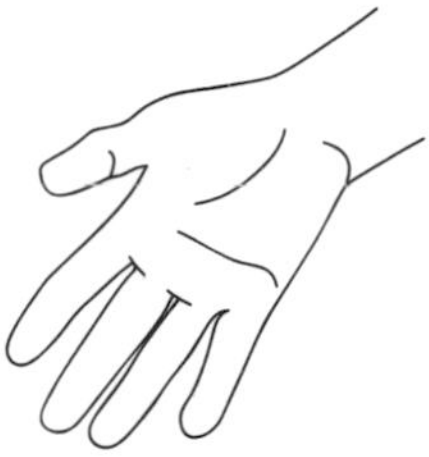

yoni-mudrā योनिमुद्रा "womb gesture"

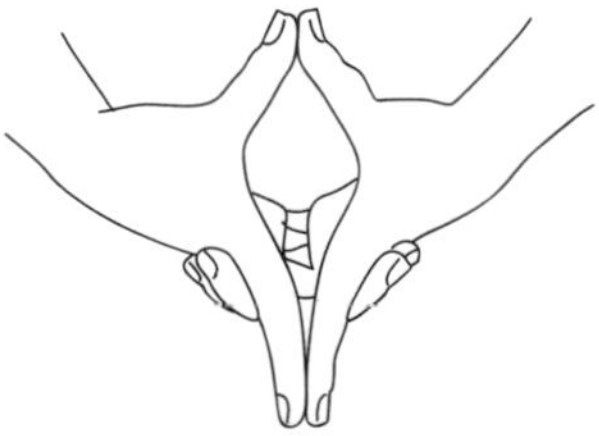

Numbers

One through twenty are commonly used by yoga practitioners, either for counting postures in a sequential flow like the sun salutation, or as part of a posture name, usually indicating how many legs or limbs are involved (eka-pāda, dvi-pāda, catuṣ-pāda).

(Note: One through four are different if declined in the neuter gender. See Āsana Names—Aṣṭāṅga Sun Salutations.)

DISC 1, TRACK 22

eka	एक	one	ekādaśa	एकादश	eleven
dvi	द्वि	two	dvādaśa	द्वादश	twelve
tri	त्रि	three	trayodaśa	त्रयोदश	thirteen
catur	चतुर्	four	caturdaśa	चतुर्दश	fourteen
pañca	पञ्च	five	pañcadaśa	पञ्चदश	fifteen
ṣaṭ	षट्	six	ṣoḍaśa	षोडश	sixteen
sapta	सप्त	seven	saptadaśa	सप्तदश	seventeen
aṣṭa/aṣṭau	अष्ट/अष्टौ	eight	aṣṭādaśa	अष्टादश	eighteen
nava	नव	nine	navadaśa	नवदश	nineteen
daśa	दश	ten	ekonaviṃśati	एकोनविंशति	nineteen
			viṃśati	विंशति	twenty

Prāṇāyāma (breath regulation)

This fourth limb of yoga involves various breathing techniques to purify the mind and strengthen the subtle energy channels (nāḍīs).

DISC 1, TRACK 23

anuloma	अनुलोम	in the natural order/direction, "with the hair"
viloma	विलोम	against the natural order/direction, "against the hair"
pratiloma	प्रतिलोम	opposite the natural order/direction, "opposite the hair"
bhastrikā	भस्त्रिका	forceful inhale and exhale, "bellows"
kapāla-bhāti	कपालभाति	breath of fire, "skull-shining"
kumbhaka	कुम्भक	breath suspension, "jar,pot"
nāḍī-śodhana	नाडीशोधन	nāḍī (energy channel) purifying
pūraka	पूरक	inhalation, "filling"
recaka	रेचक	exhalation, "emptying"
śītalī	शीतली	curl the sides of the tongue up, "cooling"
candra-bhedana	चन्द्रभेदन	left inhale, right exhale, "moon-division," cooling
sūrya-bhedana	सूर्यभेदन	right inhale, left exhale, "sun-division," heating
ujjāyī	उज्जायी	breathe making a sound in the throat by narrowing the trachea, "overcoming"

Ṣaṭ-Karmas (six cleansing actions)

The *Ṣaṭ-Karmas* are bodily cleansing techniques found in the Haṭha Yoga Pradīpikā, meant to purify the body and mind. These should only be learned from a skilled and experienced teacher.

DISC 1, TRACK 24

dhauti	धौति	swallowing cloth to clean stomach
basti	बस्ति	Āyurvedic enema
neti	नेति	nasal/sinus cleansing
trāṭaka	त्राटक	concentrated gazing
nauli	नौलि	abdominal massage
kapāla-bhāti	कपालभाति	skull-cleansing

Texts

Listed here are the major texts relating to yoga, all written in Sanskrit. The *Bhagavad-Gītā* is part of the *Mahābhārata,* which, along with the *Rāmāyaṇa,* comprise the two gigantic Indian epics.

DISC 1, TRACK 25

Bhagavad-Gītā	भगवद्गीता	conversation between Kṛṣṇa (God) and Arjuna (human), "divine song"
Gheraṇḍa Samhitā	घेरण्ड संहिता	treatise on Haṭha Yoga
Haṭhayoga Pradīpikā	हठयोग प्रदीपिका	treatise on Haṭha Yoga, "illumination of Haṭha Yoga"
Mahābhārata	महाभारत	epic story containing the *Bhagavad-Gītā,* "great-India"
Rāmāyaṇa	रामायण	epic story about the life of Rāma, "comings and goings of Rāma"
Śiva Samhitā	शिव संहिता	treatise on Haṭha Yoga
Yoga-Darśana	योगदर्शन	Yoga Sūtras by Patañjali
Yoga-Vasiṣṭha	योगवसिष्ठ	treatise on yoga

Upaniṣads

The *Upaniṣads* are the source of *Vedānta* philosophy. The thirteen texts discussed here are the most common. They are extrapolations and encapsulations of the Vedas and shared with a student who was sitting (*ṣad*), near (*upa*), and beneath (*ni*) the teacher.

DISC 1, TRACK 26

Aitareya	ऐतरेय	name of a sage
Bṛhad-Āraṇyaka	बृहदारण्यक	great forest
Chāndogya	छान्दोग्य	named after part of the Veda
Īśā	ईशा	lord
Kaṭha	कठ	named after part of the Yajur Veda
Kauṣītaki	कौषीतकि	name of sage who taught it
Kena	केन	by whom?
Maitri	मैत्रि	friendship
Māṇḍūkya	माण्डूक्य	name of sage who taught it
Muṇḍaka	मुण्डक	shaved
Praśna	प्रश्न	question
Śvetāśvatara	श्वेताश्वतर	white horse
Taittirīya	तैत्तिरीय	named after part of the Yajur Veda

Vāyus (winds of the body)

Vāyus are the primary components of breath. These energies are responsible for all movement in the body. Governed by *prāṇa*, all five affect and are affected by an āsana.

DISC 1, TRACK 27

apāna	अपान	downward moving force governing excretion, "downward breath"
prāṇa	प्राण	primary moving force governing ingestion, attention, "primary breath"
samāna	समान	inward moving force governing digestion and homeostasis, "equalizing breath"
vyāna	व्यान	outward moving force governing circulation, "pervading breath"
udāna	उदान	upward moving force governing effort, speech, "upward breath"

Vedas

Vedas are the original Sanskrit texts, forming the foundation of Indian philosophy and yoga. All are written in poetic verse and have been chanted for generations since at least 1500 BCE.

DISC 1, TRACK 28

Ṛg Veda	ऋग्वेद्	the first Veda, source of mantras
Sāma Veda	सामवेद्	the second Veda, singing of mantras
Yajur Veda	यजुर्वेद्	the third Veda, application of mantras in ritual
Atharva Veda	अथर्ववेद्	the fourth Veda, supplementary Vedic mantras

General Yoga Terms

DISC 1, TRACK 29

abhyāsa	अभ्यास	practice, focus
advaita	अद्वैत	non-duality principle
agni	अग्नि	fire principle
ahaṅkāra	अहङ्कार	ego, "I the doer"
ālamba	आलम्ब	support
ānanda	आनन्द्	joyfulness
aṣṭāṅga	अष्टाङ्ग	eight-limbs of yoga (see Aṣṭāṅga section)
ātman	आत्मन्	soul, self
Āyurveda	आयुर्वेद्	science of life/longevity, 5000-year-old holistic system of medicine from India
baddha	बद्ध	bound
bandha	बन्ध	a binding, lock (see Bandhas)
bhakti	भक्ति	devotion
bhāvana	भावन	intention, attitude
bhūmi	भूमि	earth
bhūta	भूत	element (see Elements)
buddhi	बुद्धि	intellect, reason, decision-making aspect of the citta
cakra	चक्र	energy center in the subtle body, "wheel" (see Cakras)
candra	चन्द्र	moon
cikitsā	चिकित्सा	treatment, therapy

cit	चित्	pure consciousness (without *guṇas*)
citta	चित्त	conditioned consciousness (with guṇas)
daṇḍa	दण्ड	staff, pole
deva	देव	God, male deity (see Deities and Sages)
devī	देवी	Goddess, female deity (see Deities and Sages)
dhanur	धनुर्	bow
dharma	धर्म	religion, law, duty, virtue, that which upholds
dṛṣṭi	दृष्टि	view (see Dṛṣṭis)
duḥkha	दुःख	pain, suffering "bad space"
ekāgratā	एकाग्रता	one-pointedness
guru	गुरु	teacher
guṇa	गुण	attribute, quality (see sattva, rajas, tamas)
haṭha	हठ	force, joining of sun (*ha*) and moon (*ṭha*)
hṛdaya	हृदय	heart
iḍā	इडा	left nāḍī (feminine, lunar)
indriya	इन्द्रिय	sense-organ (eye, ear, nose, tongue, skin)
Īśvara	ईश्वर	personal God
jīvātman	जीवात्मन्	individual-self enshrined in the human body
jñāna	ज्ञान	knowledge, insight
kanda	कन्द	knot
karma	कर्म	action, effect of past actions
karuṇā	करुणा	compassion
kīrtana	कीर्तन	telling, praising

General Yoga Terms (continued)

kleśa	क्लेश	affliction (see Kleśas)
koṇa	कोण	angle
kriyā	क्रिया	action, work
kuṇḍalinī	कुण्डलिनी	energy which moves up the body through the suṣumnā nāḍī "having a coil"
laghu	लघु	light-weight
liṅga	लिङ्ग	phallic symbol of Śiva, subtle body, "mark"
madhya	मध्य	middle
mālā	माला	garland, necklace
maṇḍala	मण्डल	circle
mantra	मन्त्र	sacred sound
mokṣa	मोक्ष	liberation, freedom
mudrā	मुद्रा	seal, gesture (see Mudrās)
mukta	मुक्त	released, liberated, freed
mūla	मूल	root, foundation
muni	मुनि	sage
nāḍī	नाडी	channel through which energy travels
nāga	नाग	snake
namaskāra	नमस्कार	a very respectful greeting
namaste	नमस्ते	a greeting, "salutations to you"
nātha	नाथ	yogic lineage
nidrā	निद्रा	deep, dreamless sleep, fourth *vṛtti*
nirodha	निरोध	stilling, restraint, thinning out, cessation

nirvāṇa	निर्वाण	extinguishing, liberated from existence, "without wind" or "blown out"
ojas	ओजस्	strength of prāṇa, subtle energy of the immune system
padma	पद्म	lotus
paramātman	परमात्मन्	higher-Self, supreme-Self
pariṇāma	परिणाम	transformation, change
paripūrṇa	परिपूर्ण	entire
piṅgalā	पिङ्गला	right nāḍī (masculine, solar)
prakṛti	प्रकृति	manifest world, nature, one's genetic constitution
prajñā	प्रज्ञा	insight, wisdom
prāṇa	प्राण	breath, energy (see Vāyus)
prāṇāyāma	प्राणायाम	breath regulation (see Prāṇāyāma)
pūjā	पूजा	worshipful celebration
puruṣa	पुरुष	witnessing consciousness unaffected by the material world
rāja	राज	king
rajas	रजस्	guṇa of activity
rūpa	रूप	form
śakti	शक्ति	power, ability, energy, name of Śiva's consort
sama	सम	equal, same
saṃsāra	संसार	perpetual cycle of birth and death
saṃskāra	संस्कार	acquired subliminal impressions, habits

samyama	संयम	complete control (of the mind); the last three limbs of yoga
śānti	शान्ति	peace, calmness
sarva	सर्व	all
ṣaṭ-karma	षट्कर्म	six (cleansing) actions (see Ṣaṭ-Karmas)
sattva	सत्त्व	guṇa of light, intelligence, purity
siddha	सिद्ध	accomplished
siddhi	सिद्धि	power, accomplishment
soma	सोम	yogic nectar, sacred juice, moon
sthira	स्थिर	stable
sukha	सुख	pleasurable, comfortable, "good space"
śūnya	शून्य	empty, zero, void
śūnyatā	शून्यता	emptiness
sūrya	सूर्य	sun
suṣumnā	सुषुम्ना	central nāḍī near the spinal cord (neutral)
sūtra	सूत्र	thread, aphorism
svarūpa	स्वरूप	one's own true nature, "own-form"
tamas	तमस्	guṇa of dullness, inertia
Tantra	तन्त्र	technique usually involving mantra, yantra, and deities, especially the Goddess
tapas	तपस्	a practice causing change, "heat"
tejas	तेजस्	brilliance and heat of prāṇa, fire (see Elements)
ubhaya	उभय	both

upaniṣad	उपनिषद्	texts compiled after the Vedas encapsulating their wisdom, "sitting close and beneath," (see Upaniṣads)
vāc	वाच्	speech
vairāgya	वैराग्य	non-attached awareness
vajra	वज्र	hard, diamond, thunderbolt
vāsanā	वासना	innate predisposition, tendency, trait
vastu	वस्तु	object, design, science of placing objects
vāyu	वायु	wind (see Vāyus)
veda	वेद	knowledge, name of ancient Indian scriptures (see Vedas)
Vedānta	वेदान्त	philosophy of Vedic thought encapsulated in the Upaniṣads, "essence of the Vedas"
viniyoga	विनियोग	application of yoga
vinyāsa	विन्यास	flowing sequence, arrangement
vīrya	वीर्य	strength, virility
viṣaya	विषय	object of the senses
vṛtti	वृत्ति	fluctuation, activity, "a turning"
yantra	यन्त्र	visual geometrical pattern
yoga	योग	union, connection, relationship

Aṣṭāṅga Sequences

There are six "series" of postures in this system of yoga, each one a prerequisite for the next, and each gradually increasing in level of difficulty.

Very few practitioners go beyond the third series. The sequences are characterized by a *vinyāsa* style, practicing the postures continuously from start to finish, using the breath to count holds, and moving from one pose to another on each inhalation or exhalation.

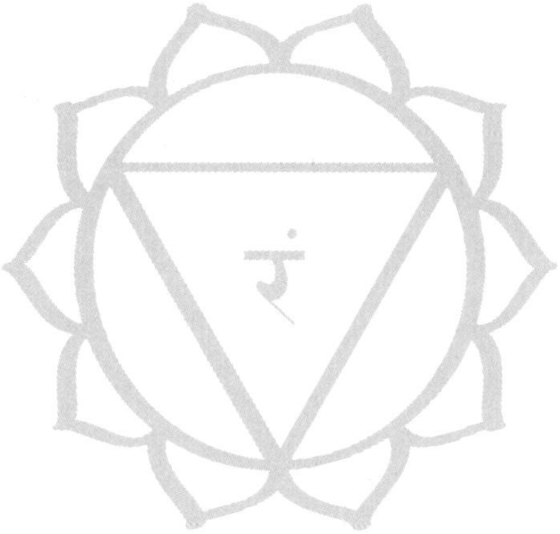

The first-series section takes a practitioner through the entire primary series, including the invocation chant. The second and third series show only the core postures for each. To go through the entire second or third series, simply replace the "seated postures" section of the first series with the core postures shown in the second or third series.

AṢṬĀṄGA FIRST SERIES

Yoga Cikitsā

Yoga Therapeutics

योगचिकित्सा

Invocation Chant: Vande Gurūṇām

DISC 2, TRACK 1

Devotion to the lotus feet of all gurus, equated with Śiva. Second half to Patañjali, considered an incarnation of Viṣṇu.

वन्दे गुरूणां चरणारविन्दे	vande gurūṇāṃ caraṇāravinde
संदर्शितस्वात्मसुखावबोधे ।	saṃdarśita-svātma-sukhāvabodhe,
निःश्रेयसे जाङ्गलिकायमाने	niḥśreyase jāṅgalikāyamāne
संसारहालाहलमोहशान्त्यै ॥	saṃsāra-hālāhala-moha-śāntyai.
आबाहुपुरुषाकारं	ābāhu puruṣākāraṃ
शङ्खचक्रासिधारिणम् ।	śaṅkha-cakrāsi-dhāriṇaṃ,
सहस्रशिरसं श्वेतं	sahasra-śirasaṃ śvetaṃ
प्रणमामि पतञ्जलिम् ॥	praṇamāmi Patañjalim.

I worship the lotus feet of all the gurus,
which awaken and manifest joy in oneself;
beyond comparison, appearing as a snake-charmer (Śiva)
for pacifying the poisonous delusion of saṃsāra (the cycle of birth and death).

In the form of a man up to the shoulders,
holding the conch (divine sound), discus (wheel of time),
and sword (discrimination),
thousand-headed, white,
I bow respectfully to Patañjali.

Sun Salutations

All three Aṣṭāṅga series begin with Sun Salutations and Standing Postures.

Sūrya-Namaskāra Ka
Sun-Salutation A

सूर्यनमस्कार क

DISC 2, TRACK 2

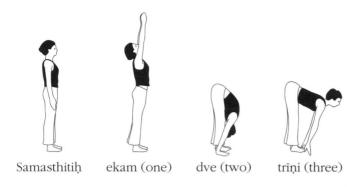

Samasthitiḥ

ekam (one)

dve (two)

trīṇi (three)

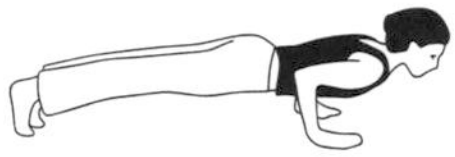
catvāri (four)

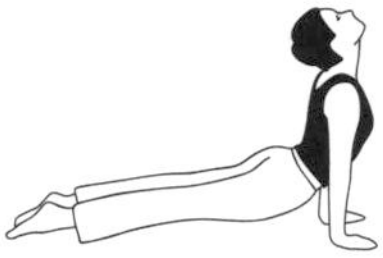
pañca (five)

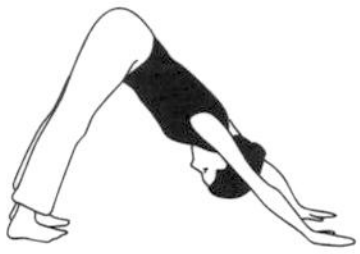
ṣaṭ (six), 5 breaths

sapta (seven)

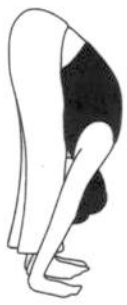
aṣṭau (eight)

nava (nine)

Samasthitiḥ

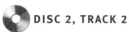

Sūrya-Namaskāra Kha

Sun-Salutation B

सूर्यनमस्कार ख

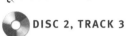

DISC 2, TRACK 3

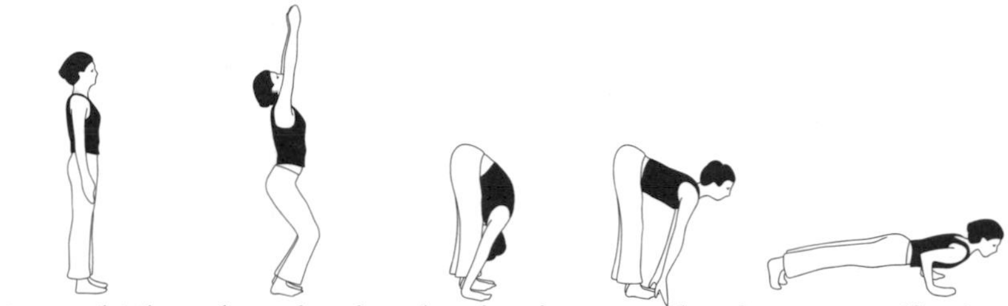

Samasthitiḥ ekam (one) dve (two) trīṇi (three) catvāri (four)

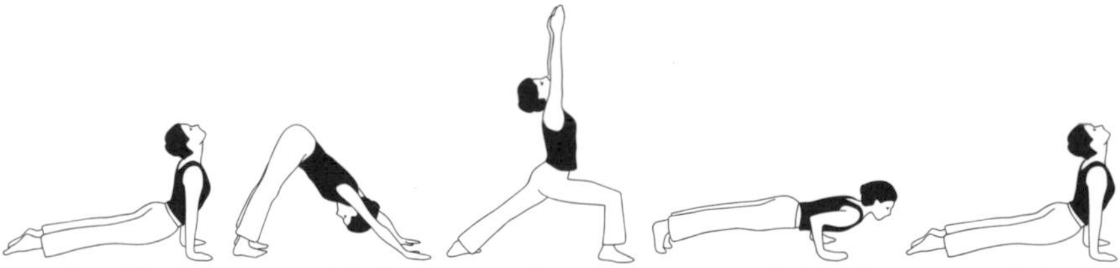

pañca (five) ṣaṭ (six) sapta (seven) aṣṭau (eight) nava (nine)

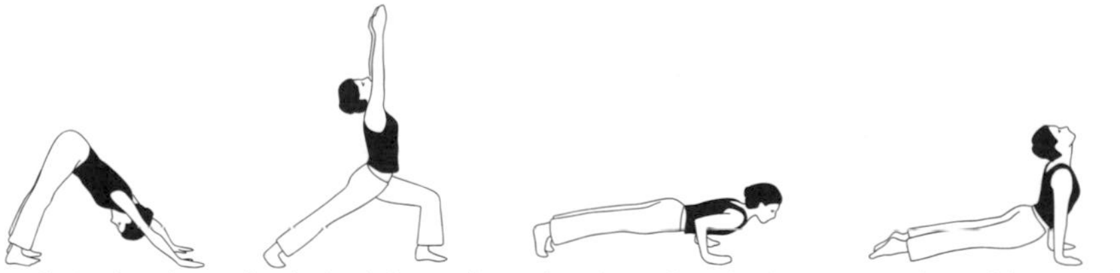

daśa (ten) ekādaśa (eleven) dvādaśa (twelve) trayodaśa (thirteen)

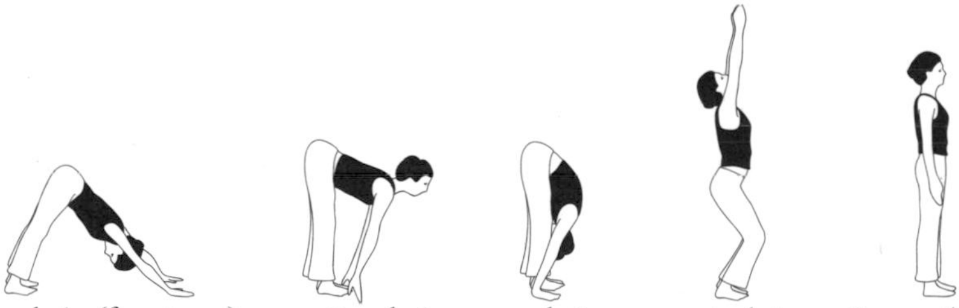

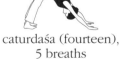

caturdaśa (fourteen), 5 breaths pañcadaśa (fifteen) ṣoḍaśa (sixteen) saptadaśa (seventeen) Samasthitiḥ

Standing Postures

DISC 2, TRACK 4
Find individual postures with the time points provided.

:03

Samasthitiḥ
Equal standing
समस्थितिः

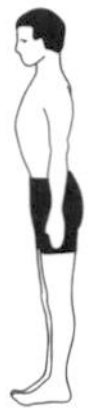

:06

1

Pādāṅguṣṭhāsana
Big toe posture
पादाङ्गुष्ठासन

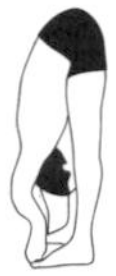

:11

2

Pāda-Hastāsana
Foot-hand posture
पादहस्तासन

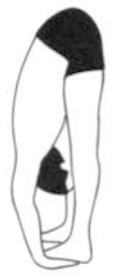

:16

3

Utthita-Trikoṇāsana (ka, kha)
Extended triangle posture (a, b)
उत्थितत्रिकोणासन (क ख)

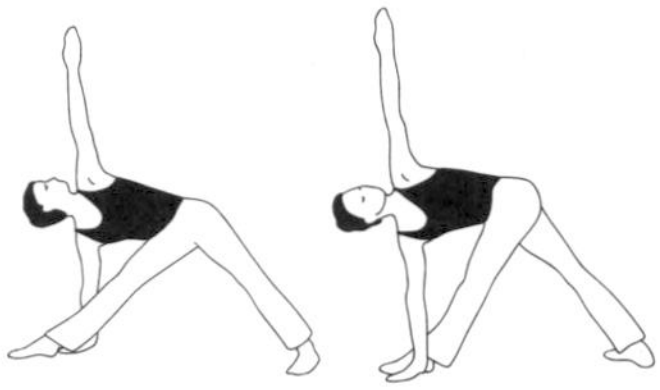

:25

4

Utthita-Pārśvakoṇāsana
Extended side-angle posture
उत्थितपार्श्वकोणासन

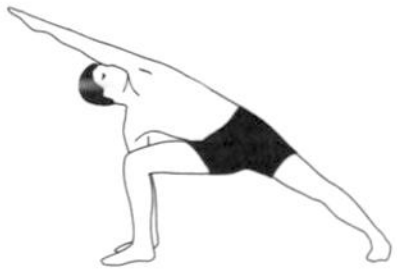

:32

5

Prasārita-Pādottānāsana (ka, kha, ga, gha)
Spread-leg stretched-out posture (a, b, c, d)
प्रसारितपादोत्तानासन (क ख ग घ)

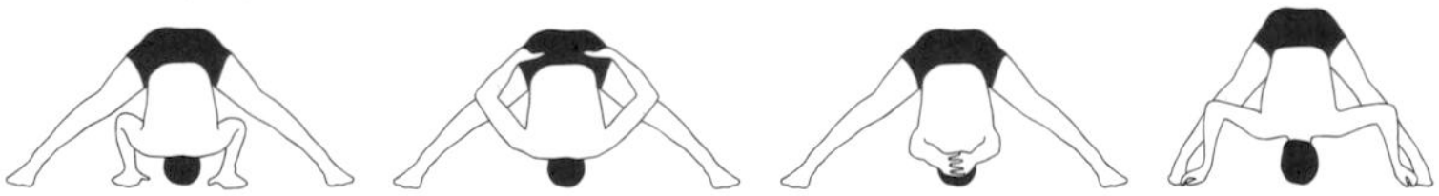

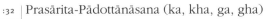

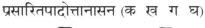

:46 | Pārśvottānāsana

6 Side-stretched out posture

पार्श्वोत्तानासन

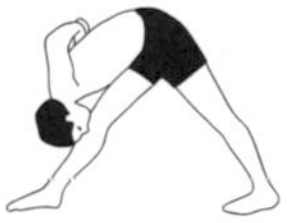

:52 | Utthita-Hasta-Pādāṅguṣṭhāsana

7 Extended hand-foot-big toe posture

उत्थितहस्तपादाङ्गुष्ठासन

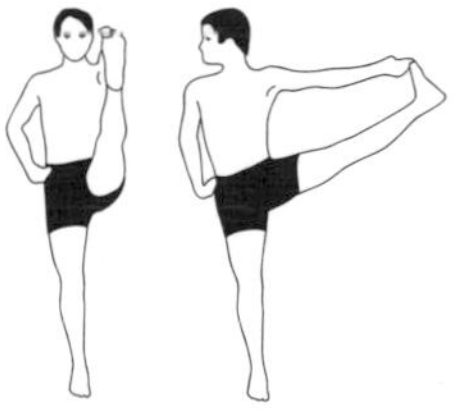

1:01 | Ardha-Baddha-Padmottānāsana

8 Half-bound lotus stretched-out posture

अर्धबद्धपद्मोत्तानासन

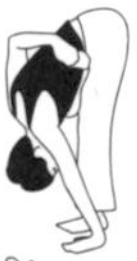

1:09 | Utkaṭāsana

9 Mighty posture

उत्कटासन

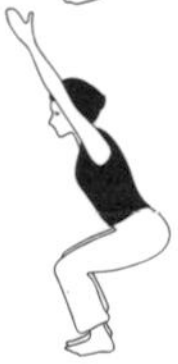

1:14 | Vīrabhadrāsana (ka, kha)

10 Warrior posture (a, b)

वरिभद्रासन (क ख)

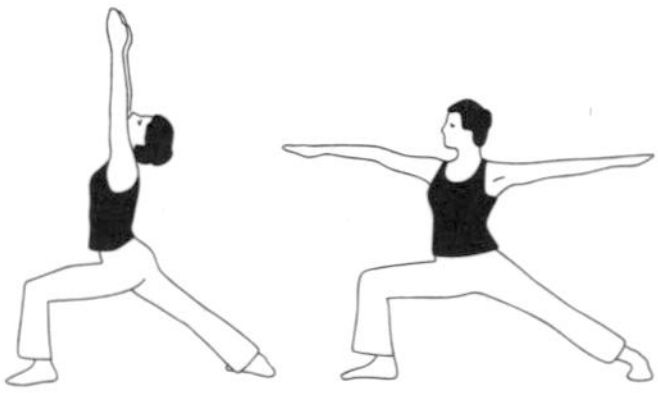

Seated Postures

DISC 2, TRACK 5
Find individual postures with the time points provided.

* Indicates a transition posture that is not specifically named in the traditional sequence. Most have no numbers.

:03
Daṇḍāsana *
Staff posture
दण्डासन

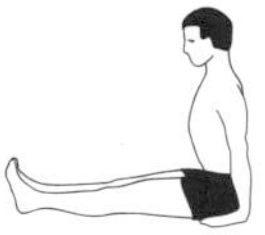

:07
11
Paścimatānāsana
Back stretched-out posture
पश्चिमतानासन

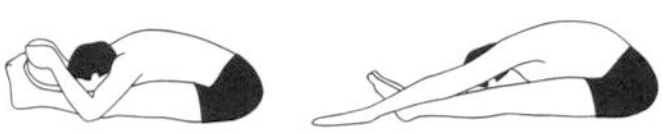

:12
12
Pūrvatānāsana
Front stretched-out posture
पूर्वतानासन

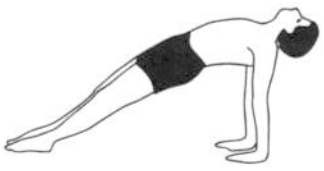

:17
13
Ardha-Baddha-Padma-Paścimatānāsana
Half-bound lotus
back stretched-out posture
अर्धबद्धपद्मपश्चिमतानासन

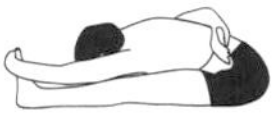

:27
14
Tiryaṅ-Mukhaikapāda-Paścimatānāsana
Oblique face one-leg-back
stretched-out posture
तिर्यङ्मुखैकपादपश्चिमतानासन

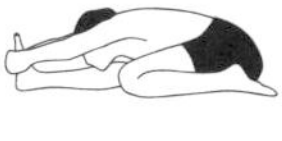

:37
15
Jānu-Śīrṣāsana (ka, kha, ga)
Knee-head posture (a, b, c)
जानुशीर्षासन (क ख ग)

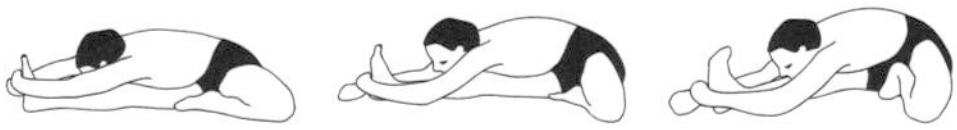

:47 Marīcyāsana (ka, kha, ga, gha)

16 Marīci (son of Brahma) posture (a, b, c, d)

मरीच्यासन (क ख ग घ)

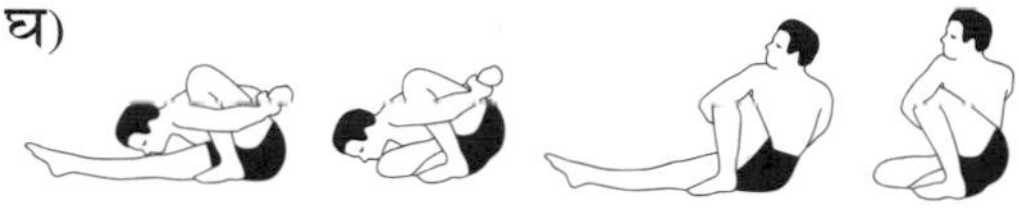

:59 Nāvāsana

17 Boat posture

नावासन

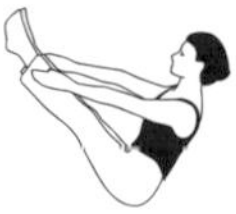

1:03 Bhuja-Pīḍāsana

18 Arm-pressure posture

भुजपीडासन

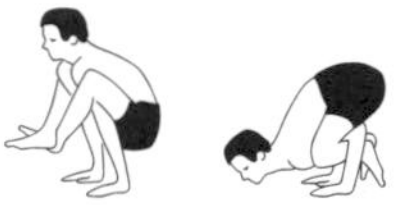

1:09 Kūrmāsana

19 Tortoise posture

कूर्मासन

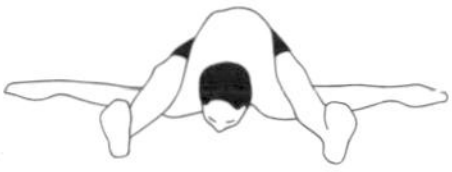

1:13 Supta-Kūrmāsana

20 Supine-tortoise posture

सुप्तकूर्मासन

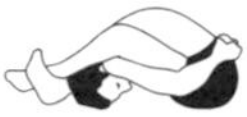

1:17 Garbha-Piṇḍāsana

21 Womb-ball posture

गर्भपिण्डासन

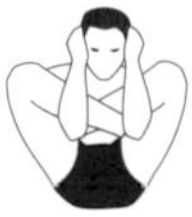

1:22 Kukkuṭāsana

22 Rooster posture

कुक्कुटासन

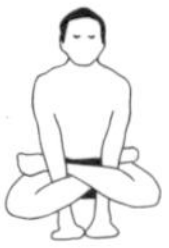

1:26 Baddha-Koṇāsana

23 Bound-angle posture

बद्धकोणासन

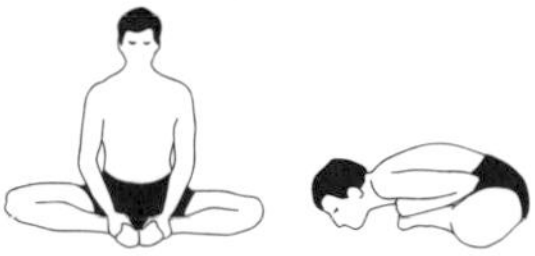

Seated Postures (continued)

1:32 | **24** | Upaviṣṭa-Koṇāsana
Seated-angle posture
उपविष्टकोणासन

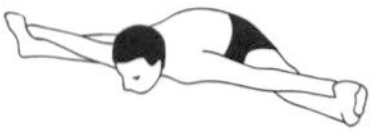

1:37 | **25** | Supta-Koṇāsana
Supine-angle posture
सुPकोणासन

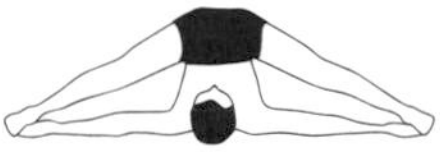

1:42 | **26** | Supta-Pādāṅguṣṭhāsana
supine-big toe posture
सुPपादाङ्गुष्ठासन

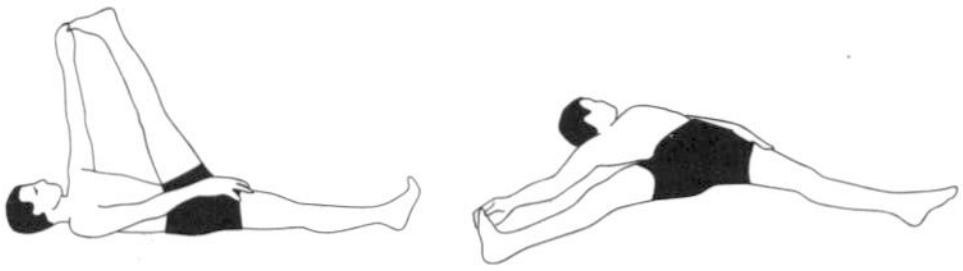

1:48 | **27** | Ubhaya-Pādāṅguṣṭhāsana
Both-feet big-toe posture
उभयपादाङ्गुष्ठासन

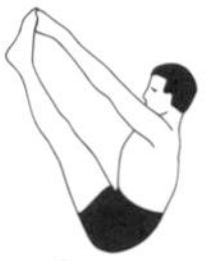

1:56 | **28** | Ūrdhva-Mukha-Paścimottānāsana
Upward-facing back-stretched out posture
ऊर्ध्वमुखपश्चिमोत्तानासन

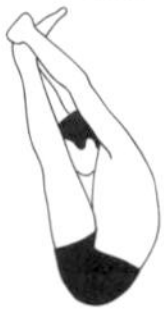

2:03 | **29** | Setu-Bandhāsana
Bridge-building posture
सेतुबन्धासन

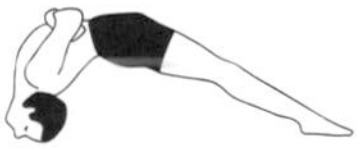

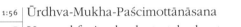

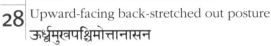

Finishing Postures

DISC 2, TRACK 6
Find individual postures with the time points provided.

All three Aṣṭāṅga series end with these postures.

* Indicates a transition posture that is not specifically named in the traditional sequence. Most have no numbers.

:02
Ūrdhva-Dhanurāsana *
Upward bow posture
ऊर्ध्वधनुरासन

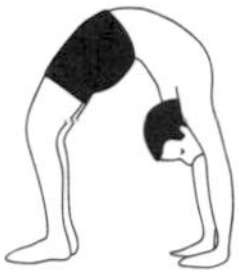

:07
Paścimatānāsana *
Back stretched-out posture
पश्चिमतानासन

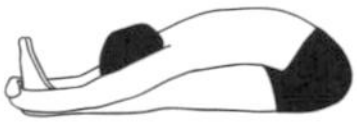

:12
30
Sarvāṅgāsana
All-limb posture
सर्वाङ्गासन

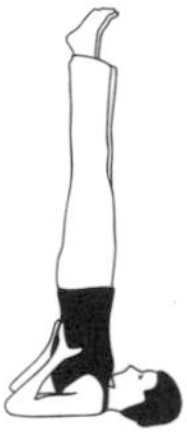

:17
31
Halāsana
Plow posture
हलासन

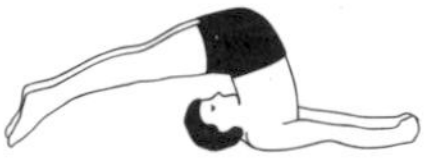

:20
32
Karṇa-Pīḍāsana
Ear-pressure posture
कर्णपीडासन

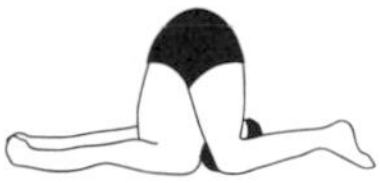

:25
33
Ūrdhva-Padmāsana
Upward-lotus posture
ऊर्ध्वपद्मासन

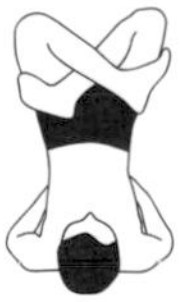

:30
34
Piṇḍāsana
Ball posture
पिण्डासन

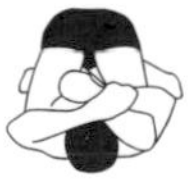

Finishing Postures (continued)

:34 Matsyāsana

35 Fish posture

मत्स्यासन

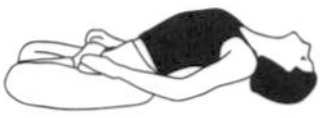

:38 Uttāna-Pādāsana

36 Stretched-out leg posture

उत्तानपादासन

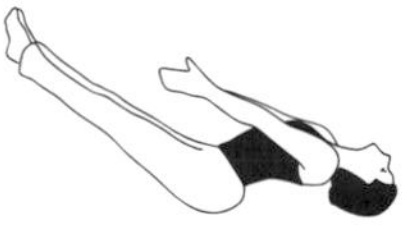

:43 Cakrāsana *

Wheel posture

चक्रासन

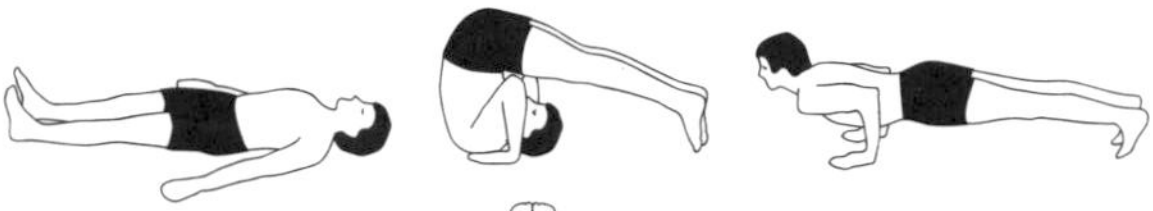

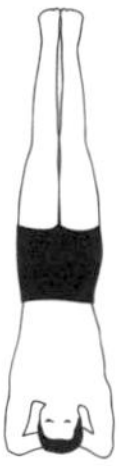

:47 Śīrṣāsana

37 Head posture

शीर्षासन

:51 Baddha-Padmāsana

38 Bound-lotus posture

बद्धपद्मासन

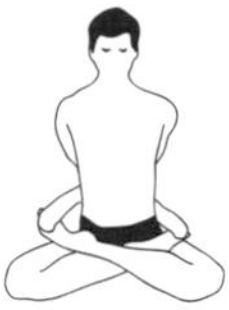

:56 Yoga-Mudrā (part of Baddha-Padmāsana)

Yoga seal

योगमुद्रा

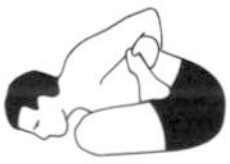

1:00 Padmāsana

39 Lotus posture

पद्मासन

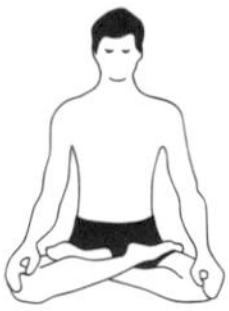

1:04 Utplutiḥ

40 Upward floating

उत्प्लुतिः

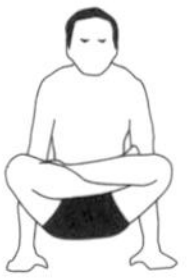

Prathamo bhāgaḥ samāptaḥ
First Part Finished

प्रथमो भागः समाप्तः

Aṣṭāṅga First Series Summary

SUN SALUTATIONS		PAGE
	Sūrya-Namaskāra Ka	46
	Sūrya-Namaskāra Kha	47

STANDING POSTURES		PAGE
	Samasthitiḥ	48
1	Pādāṅguṣṭhāsana	48
2	Pāda-Hastāsana	48
3	Utthita-Trikoṇāsana (ka,kha)	48
4	Utthita-Pārśvakoṇāsana	48
5	Prasārita-Pādottānāsana (ka, kha, ga, gha)	48
6	Pārśvottānāsana	49
7	Utthita-Hasta-Pādāṅguṣṭhāsana	49
8	Ardha-Baddha-Padmottānāsana	49
9	Utkaṭāsana	
10	Vīrabhadrāsana (ka, kha)	49

SEATED POSTURES		PAGE
	Daṇḍāsana *	50
11	Paścimatānāsana	50
12	Pūrvatānāsana	50
13	Ardha-Baddha-Padma-Paścimatānāsana	50
14	Tiryaṅ-Mukhaikapāda-Paścimatānāsana	50
15	Jānu-Śīrṣāsana (ka, kha, ga)	50
16	Marīcyāsana (ka, kha, ga, gha)	51
17	Nāvāsana	51
18	Bhuja-Pīḍāsana	51
19	Kūrmāsana	51
20	Supta-Kūrmāsana	51
21	Garbha-Piṇḍāsana	51
22	Kukkuṭāsana	51
23	Baddha-Koṇāsana	51
24	Upaviṣṭa-Koṇāsana	52
25	Supta-Koṇāsana	52
26	Supta-Pādāṅguṣṭhāsana	52
27	Ubhaya-Pādāṅguṣṭhāsana	52
28	Ūrdhva-Mukha-Paścimottānāsana	52
29	Setu-Bandhāsana	52

FINISHING POSTURES		PAGE
	Ūrdhva-Dhanurāsana *	53
	Paścimatānāsana *	53
30	Sarvāṅgāsana	53
31	Halāsana	53
32	Karṇa-Pīḍāsana	53
33	Ūrdhva-Padmāsana	53
34	Piṇḍāsana	53
35	Matsyāsana	54
36	Uttānapādāsana	54
	Cakrāsana *	54
37	Śīrṣāsana	54
38	Baddha-Padmāsana	54
	Yogamudrā	54
39	Padmāsana	54
40	Utplutiḥ	54

AṢṬĀṄGA SECOND SERIES

Nāḍī-Śodhana

Purification of the Channels

नाडीशोधन

DISC 2, TRACK 7
Find individual postures with the time points provided.

Preceded by Sun Salutations and Standing Postures (pages 46 to 49).

:12
1 Pāśāsana
Noose posture
पाशासन

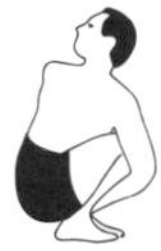

:15
2 Krauñcāsana
Heron posture
क्रौञ्चासन

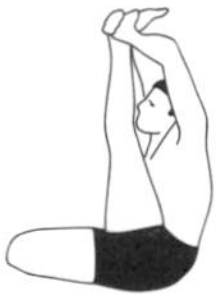

:20
3 Śalabhāsana
Locust posture
शलभासन

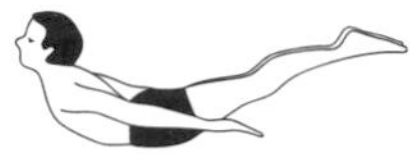

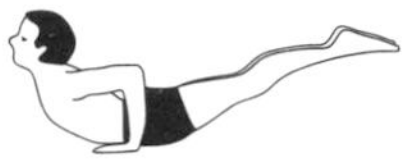

:23
4 Bhekāsana
Frog posture
भेकासन

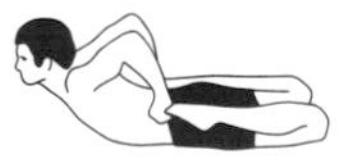

:27
5 Dhanurāsana
Bow posture
धनुरासन

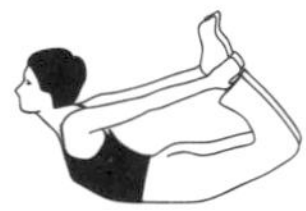

:31
6 Pārśva-Dhanurāsana
Side-bow posture
पार्श्वधनुरासन

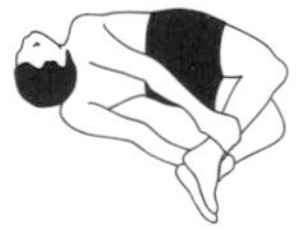

:36 Uṣṭrāsana

7 Camel posture

उष्ट्रासन

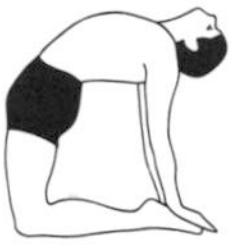

:40 Laghu-Vajrāsana

8 Light (weight) thunderbolt posture

लघुवज्रासन

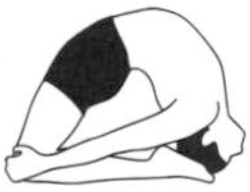

:44 Kapotāsana

9 Pigeon posture

कपोतासन

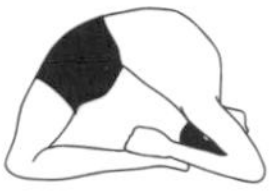

:49 Supta-Vajrāsana

10 Supine thunderbolt posture

सुप्तवज्रासन

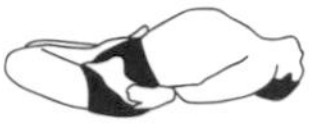

:53 Bakāsana (ka, kha)

11 Crane posture (a, b)

बकासन (क ख)

A, b entered differently but end the same

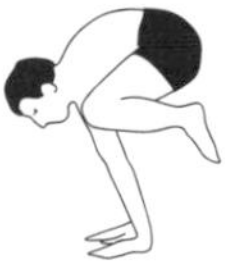

1:00 Bharadvājāsana

12 (Name of sage) posture

भरद्वाजासन

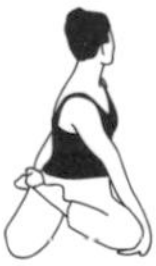

1:05 Ardha-Matsyendrāsana

13 Half-fish lord posture

अर्धमत्स्येन्द्रासन

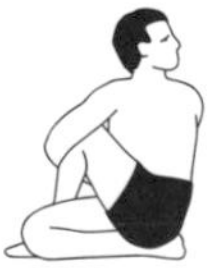

1:11 Eka-Pāda-Śīrṣāsana

14 One-leg head posture

एकपादशीर्षासन

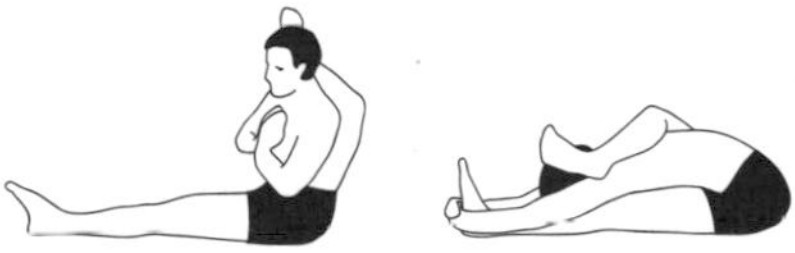

Aṣṭāṅga Second Series (continued)

15 | 1:17 Dvi-Pāda-Śīrṣāsana
Two-leg head posture
द्विपादशीर्षासन

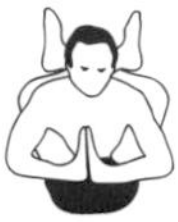

16 | 1:23 Yoga-Nidrāsana
Yoga sleep posture
योगनिद्रासन

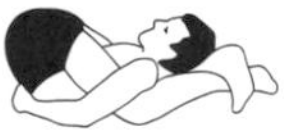

17 | 1:28 Tittibhāsana
Firefly posture
तित्तिभासन

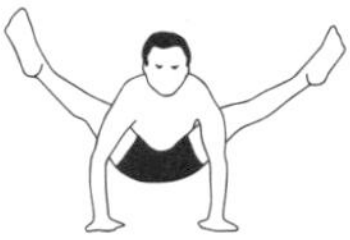

18 | 1:33 Pīñca-Mayūrāsana
Feather peacock posture
पीञ्चमयूरासन

19 | 1:38 Kāraṇḍavāsana
Himalayan goose posture
कारण्डवासन

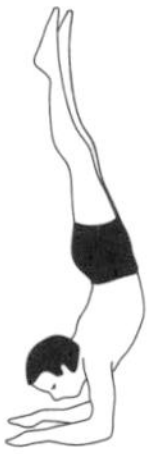

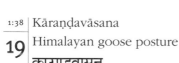

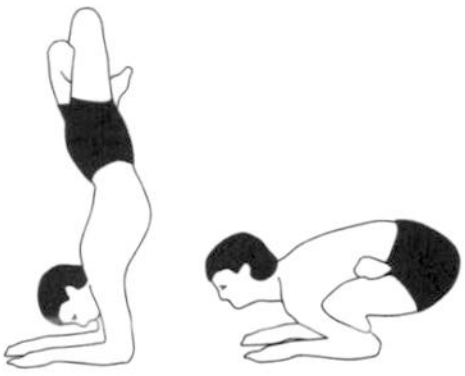

20 | 1:43 Mayūrāsana
Peacock posture
मयूरासन

21 | 1:48 Nakrāsana
Crocodile posture
नक्रासन

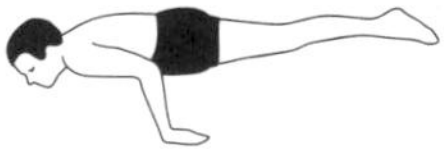

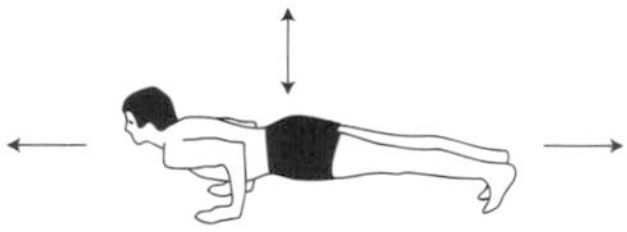

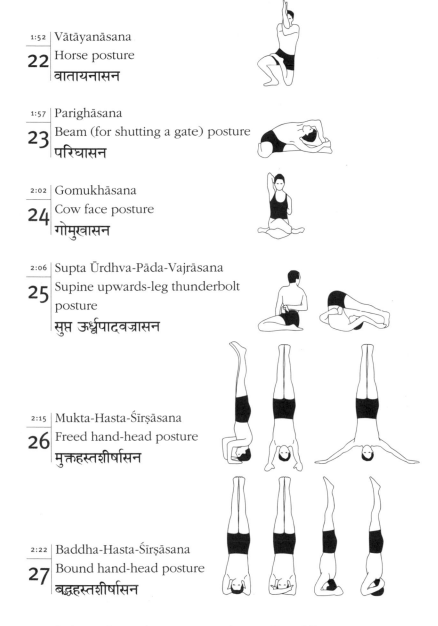

1:52 | 22 | Vātāyanāsana
Horse posture
वातायनासन

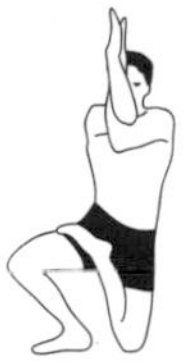

1:57 | 23 | Parighāsana
Beam (for shutting a gate) posture
परिघासन

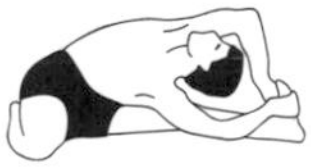

2:02 | 24 | Gomukhāsana
Cow face posture
गोमुखासन

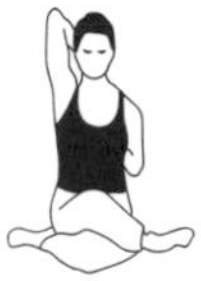

2:06 | 25 | Supta Ūrdhva-Pāda-Vajrāsana
Supine upwards-leg thunderbolt posture
सुप्त ऊर्ध्वपादवज्रासन

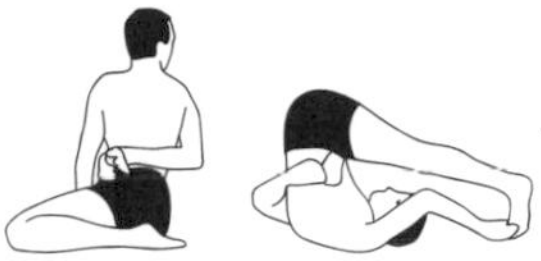

2:15 | 26 | Mukta-Hasta-Śīrṣāsana
Freed hand-head posture
मुक्तहस्तशीर्षासन

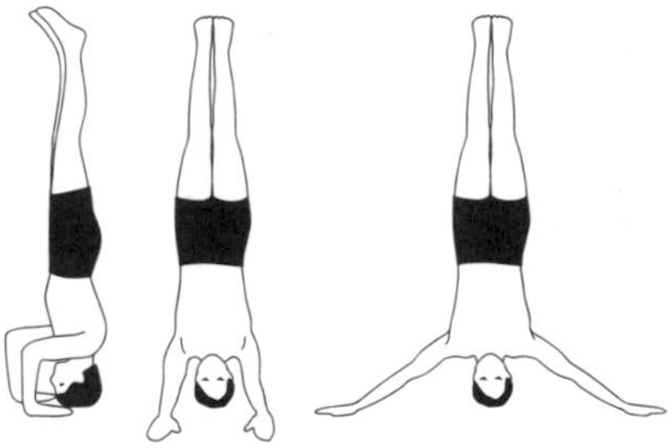

2:22 | 27 | Baddha-Hasta-Śīrṣāsana
Bound hand-head posture
बद्धहस्तशीर्षासन

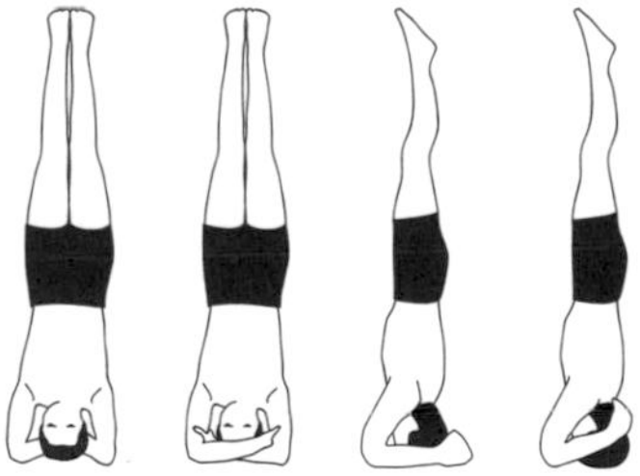

Concludes with Finishing Postures (pages 53 to 54).

Dvitīyo bhāgaḥ samāptaḥ

Second Part Finished

द्वितीयो भागः समाप्तः

Aṣṭāṅga Second Series Summary

Sun Salutations and Standing Postures same as First Series (pages 46 to 49).

		PAGE
1	Pāśāsana	56
2	Krauñcāsana	56
3	Śalabhāsana	56
4	Bhekāsana	56
5	Dhanurāsana	56
6	Pārśva-Dhanurāsana	56
7	Uṣṭrāsana	57
8	Laghu-Vajrāsana	57
9	Kapotāsana	57
10	Supta-Vajrāsana	57
11	Bakāsana (ka, kha)	57
12	Bharadvājāsana	57
13	Ardha-Matsyendrāsana	57
14	Eka-Pāda-Śīrṣāsana	57
15	Dvi-Pāda-Śīrṣāsana	58
16	Yoga-Nidrāsana	58
17	Tittibhāsana	58
18	Pīñca-Mayūrāsana	58
19	Kāraṇḍavāsana	58
20	Mayūrāsana	58
21	Nakrāsana	58
22	Vātāyanāsana	59
23	Parighāsana	59
24	Gomukhāsana	59
25	Supta Ūrdhva-Pāda-Vajrāsana	59
26	Mukta-Hasta-Śīrṣāsana	59
27	Baddha-Hasta-Śīrṣāsana	59

Finishing Postures same as First Series (pages 53 to 54).

AṢṬĀṄGA THIRD SERIES

Sthira-Bhāgaḥ
Steady Part
स्थिरभागः

DISC 2, TRACK 8
Find individual postures with the time points provided.

Preceded by Sun Salutations and Standing Postures (pages 46 to 49).

:10
1 Viśvāmitrāsana
(Name of sage) posture
विश्वामित्रासन

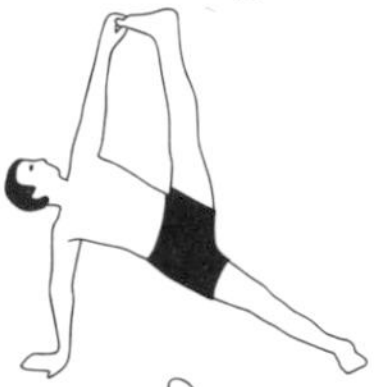

:15
2 Vasiṣṭhāsana
(Name of sage) posture
वसिष्ठासन

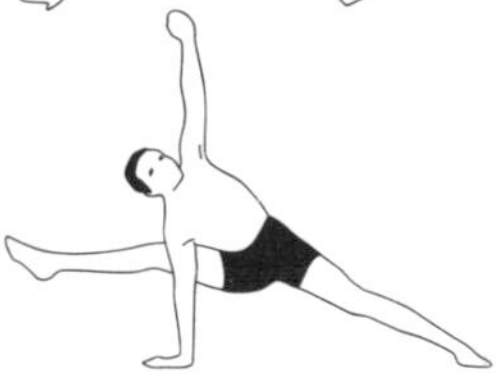

:20
3 Kaśyapāsana
(Name of sage) posture
कश्यपासन

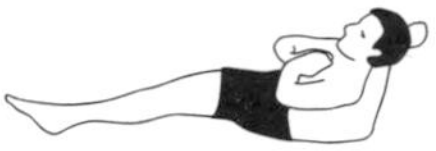

:24
4 Cakorāsana
Partridge posture
चकोरासन

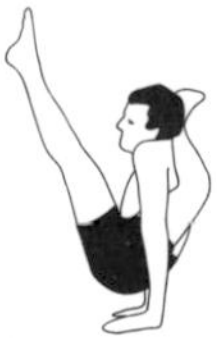

:30
5 Bhairavāsana
Formidable posture
भैरवासन

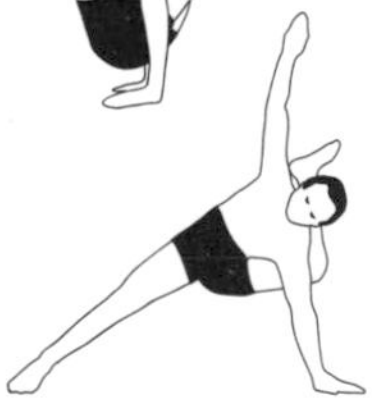

:35
6 Skandāsana
(Name of sage) posture
स्कन्दासन

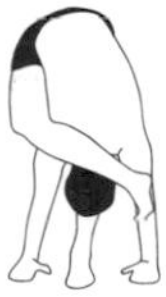

Aṣṭāṅga Third Series (continued)

:39
7
Dūrvāsāsana
(Name of sage) posture
दूर्वासासन

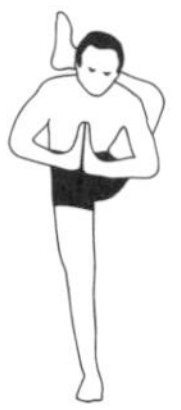

:44
8
Ūrdhva-Kukkuṭāsana (ka, kha, ga)
Upward rooster posture (a, b, c)
ऊर्ध्वकुक्कुटासन (क ख ग)
a, b, c entered differently but end the same

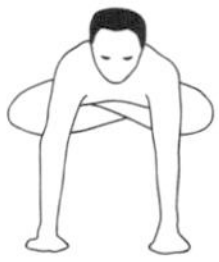

:54
9
Gālavāsana
(Name of sage) posture
गालवासन

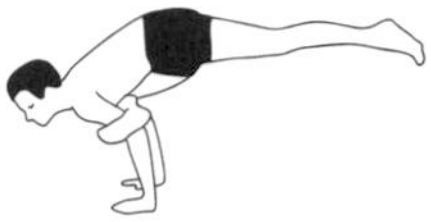

:59
10
Eka-Pāda-Bakāsana (ka, kha)
One-leg crane posture (a, b)
एकपादबकासन (क ख)

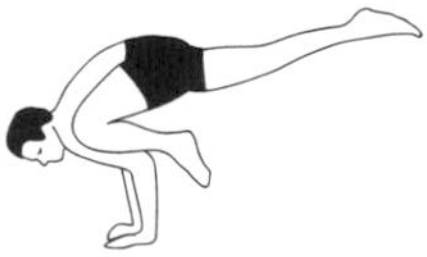
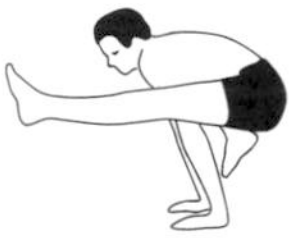

1:08
11
Kauṇḍinyāsana (ka, kha)
(Name of sage) posture (a, b)
कौण्डिन्यासन (क ख)

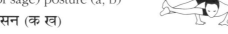

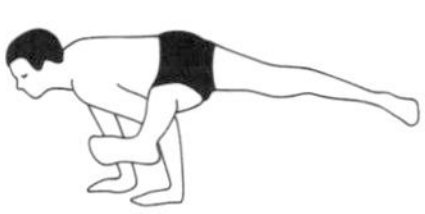
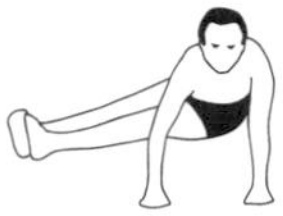

1:16
12
Aṣṭāvakrāsana (ka, kha)
(Name of sage) posture (a, b)
अष्टावक्रासन (क ख)
a, b, c entered differently but end the same

1:25
13
Paripūrṇa-Matsyendrāsana
Entire fish lord posture
परिपूर्णमत्स्येन्द्रासन

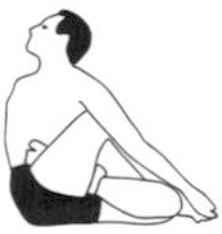

1:33 | **14** | Virañcyāsana (ka, kha)
(Name of sage) posture (a, b)
विरञ्च्यासन (क ख)

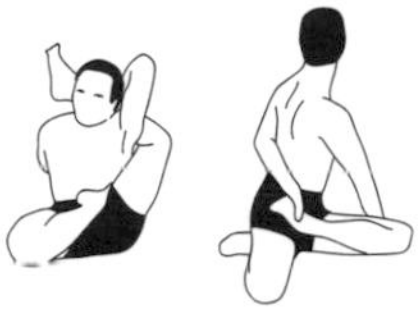

1:40 | **15** | Viparīta-Daṇḍāsana
Inverted staff posture
विपरीतदण्डासन

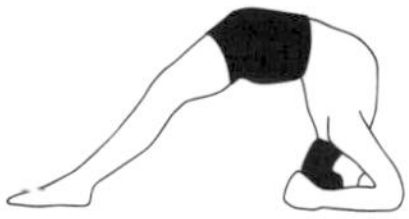

1:47 | **16** | Eka-Pāda-Viparīta-Daṇḍāsana
One-leg inverted staff posture
एकपादविपरीतदण्डासन

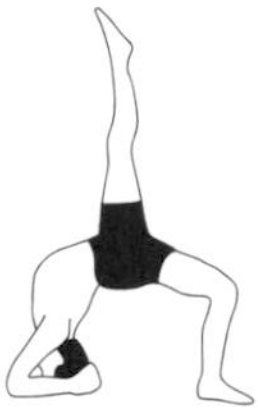

1:55 | **17** | Viparīta-Śalabhāsana
Inverted locust posture
विपरीतशलभासन

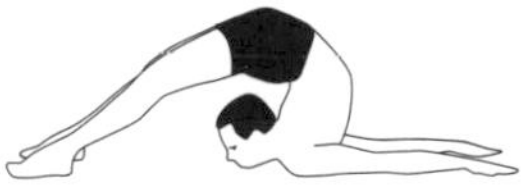

2:02 | **18** | Hanumānāsana
(Name of monkey deity) posture
हनुमानासन

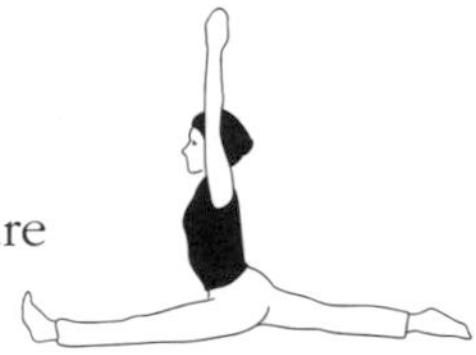

2:08 | **19** | Supta-Trivikramāsana
Supine three-stride posture
सुप्तत्रिविक्रमासन

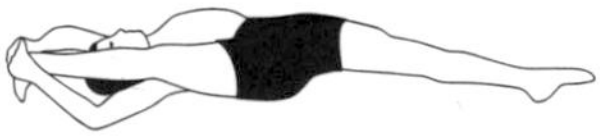

2:15 | **20** | Digāsana
Direction posture
दिगासन

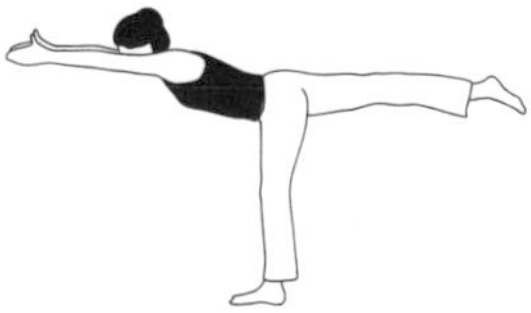

Aṣṭāṅga Third Series (continued)

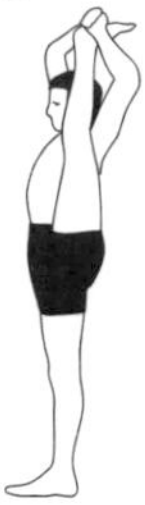

2:19 | Trivikramāsana

21 | Three-stride posture

त्रिविक्रमासन

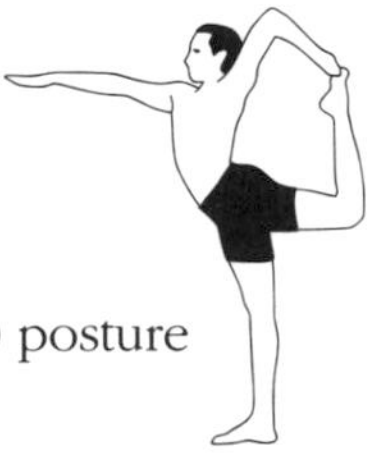

2:24 | Naṭarājāsana

22 | Lord of the dance (name of Śiva) posture

नटराजासन

2:29 | Rāja-Kapotāsana

23 | King pigeon posture

राजकपोतासन

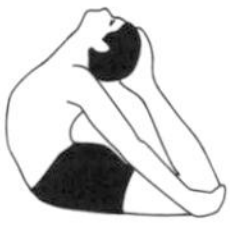

2:34 | Eka-Pāda-Rāja-Kapotāsana

24 | One-leg king pigeon posture

एकपादराजकपोतासन

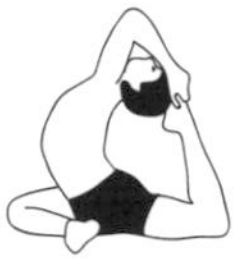

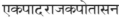

Concludes with Finishing Postures (pages 53 to 54).

Tritīyo bhāgaḥ samāptaḥ
Third Part Finished
त्रितीयो भागः समाप्तः

Aṣṭāṅga Third Series Summary

Sun Salutations and Standing Postures same as First Series (pages 46 to 49).

		PAGE
1	Viśvāmitrāsana	61
2	Vasiṣṭhāsana	61
3	Kaśyapāsana	61
4	Cakorāsana	61
5	Bhairavāsana	61
6	Skandāsana	61
7	Dūrvāsāsana	62
8	Ūrdhva-Kukkuṭāsana (ka, kha, ga)	62
9	Gālavāsana	62
10	Eka-Pāda-Bakāsana (ka, kha)	62
11	Kauṇḍinyāsana (ka, kha)	62
12	Aṣṭāvakrāsana (ka, kha)	62

		PAGE
13	Paripūrṇa-Matsyendrāsana	62
14	Virañcyāsana (ka, kha)	63
15	Viparīta-Daṇḍāsana	63
16	Eka-Pāda-Viparīta-Daṇḍāsana	63
17	Viparīta-Śalabhāsana	63
18	Hanumānāsana	63
19	Supta-Trivikramāsana	63
20	Digāsana	63
21	Trivikramāsana	64
22	Naṭarājāsana	64
23	Rāja-Kapotāsana	64
24	Eka-Pāda-Rāja-Kapotāsana	64

Finishing Postures same as First Series (pages 53 to 54).

ĀSANA NAMES

A comprehensive list of āsana names, presented in English alphabetical order and grouped by first letter.

Each name is pronounced in full twice, once at the beginning and once at the end, each time with space for you to repeat. In between, each part of the name is pronounced once, with space for you to repeat.

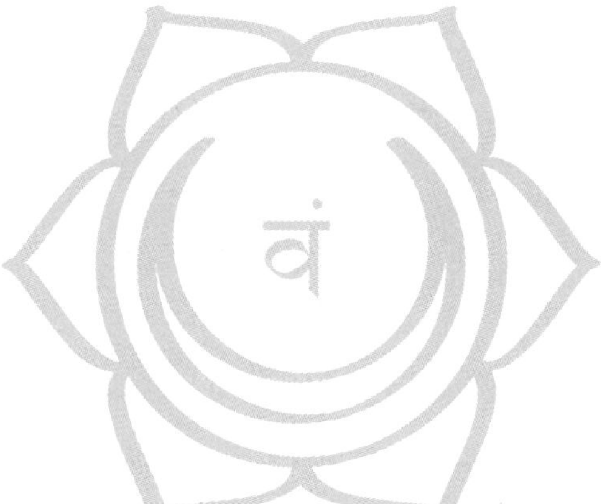

Āsana names are presented here, although not all variations are shown, due to time constraints on the CD. For each āsana, the following are shown:

UPPER LEFT CORNER: CD TIME POINT

Allows you to find the āsana name on the individual CD track. Just go to the track, then hold the fast-forward button down until you come to the time point shown.

LINE 1: FULL TRANSLITERATION

This is the full āsana name in roman letters with diacritical marks. Please see the Sanskrit Pronunciation Key in the back of the book for how to pronounce the letters.

LINE 2: SEPARATED TRANSLITERATION

So you can see each part of each word in the āsana name.

LINE 3: ENGLISH TRANSLATION

The literal meaning of the āsana name.

LINE 4: SEPARATED SANSKRIT

Sanskrit script for line 2.

LINE 5: FULL SANSKRIT

Sanskrit script for line 1. This is how you would see the āsana name in its orginal form.

RIGHT SIDE

Line drawing of the āsana, some with variations.

Note: Āsana and pīṭham both mean "posture."

A

DISC 2, TRACK 9
Find individual postures with the time points provided.

:03 Adho-Mukha-Matsyāsana
Adho - mukha - matsya - āsana
Downward - facing - fish - posture
अधो - मुख - मत्स्य - आसन
अधोमुखमत्स्यासन

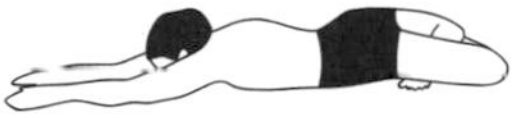

:24 Adho-Mukha-Śvānāsana
Adho - mukha - śvāna - āsana
Downward - facing - dog - posture
अधो - मुख - श्वान - आसन
अधोमुखश्वानासन

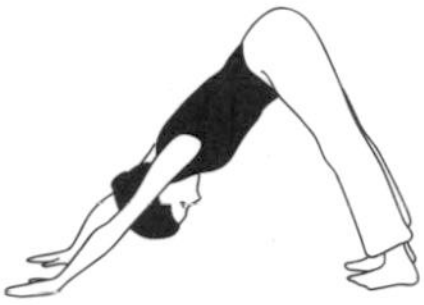

:45 Adho-Mukha-Vṛkṣāsana
Adho - mukha - vṛkṣa - āsana
Downward - facing - tree - posture
अधो - मुख - वृक्ष - आसन
अधोमुखवृक्षासन

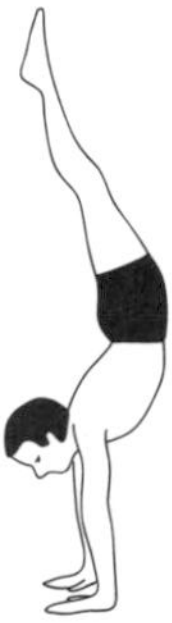

1:05 Ākarṇa-Dhanurāsana
Ā - karṇa - dhanur - āsana
Towards - ear - bow - posture
आ - कर्ण - धनुर् - आसन
आकर्णधनुरासन

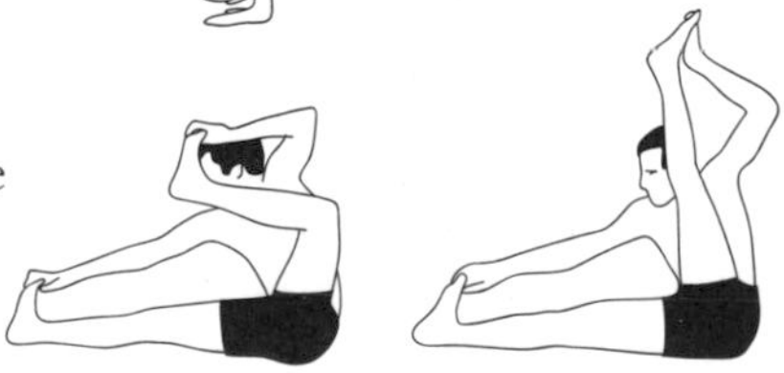

A (continued)

1:25 Ākuñcanāsana
Ākuñcana - āsana
Bending - posture
आकुञ्चन - आसन
आकुञ्चनासन

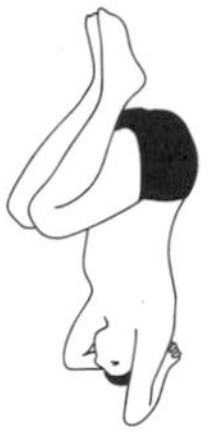

1:41 Anantāsana
Ananta - āsana
Endless (bed of Viṣṇu) - posture
अनन्त - आसन
अनन्तासन

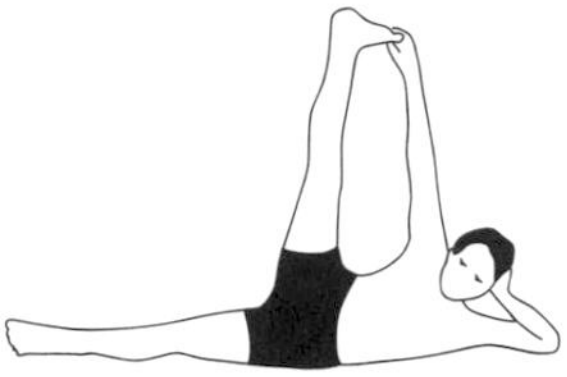

2:10 Apānāsana
Apāna - āsana
Downward air / abdominal breath - posture
अपान - आसन
अपानासन

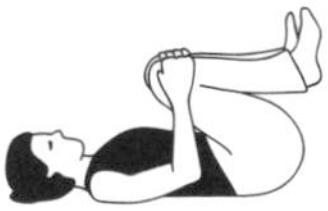

2:10 Ardha-Baddha-Padma-Paścimottānāsana
Ardha - baddha - padma - paścima - uttāna - āsana
Half - bound - lotus - back - stretched out - posture
अर्ध - बद्ध - पद्म - पश्चिम - उत्तान - आसन
अर्धबद्धपद्मपश्चिमोत्तानासन

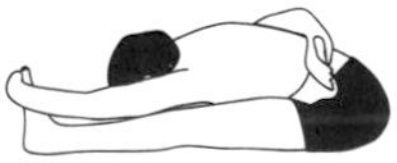

2:42 Ardha-Baddha-Padmottānāsana
Ardha - baddha - padma - uttāna - āsana
Half - bound - lotus - stretched out - posture
अर्ध - बद्ध - पद्म - उत्तान - आसन
अर्धबद्धपद्मोत्तानासन

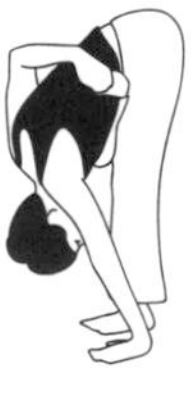

3:04 Ardha-Candrāsana
Ardha - candra - āsana
Half - moon - posture
अर्ध - चन्द्र - आसन
अर्धचन्द्रासन

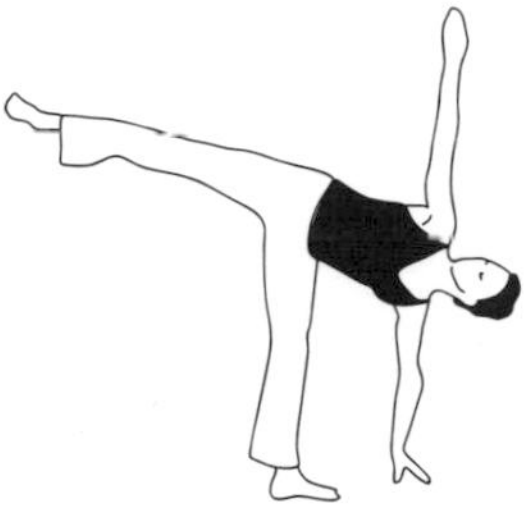

3:20 Ardha-Matsyendrāsana
Ardha - matsya - Indra - āsana
Half - fish - lord - posture
अर्ध - मत्स्य - इन्द्र - आसन
अर्धमत्स्येन्द्रासन

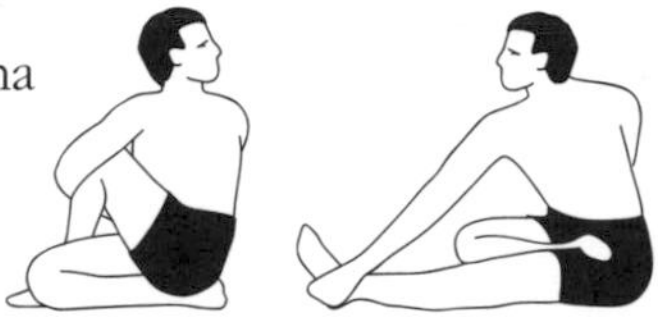

3:39 Ardha-Nāvāsana
Ardha - nāva - āsana
Half - boat - posture
अर्ध - नाव - आसन
अर्धनावासन

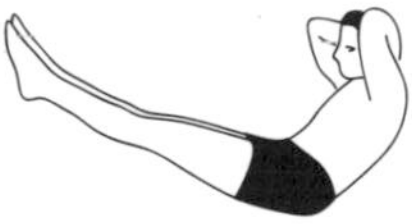

3:54 Ardha-Śalabhāsana
Ardha - śalabha - āsana
Half - locust - posture
अर्ध - शलभ - आसन
अर्धशलभासन

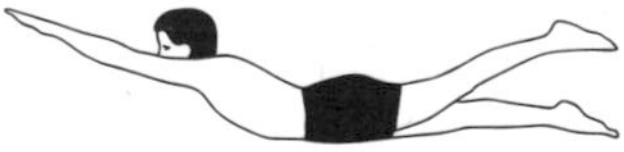

4:09 Aṣṭāvakrāsana
Aṣṭāvakra - āsana
(Name of sage) - posture
अष्टावक्र - आसन
अष्टावक्रासन

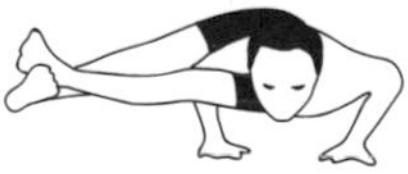

B

DISC 2, TRACK 10
Find individual postures with the time points provided.

:03 Baddha-Hasta-Śīrṣāsana
Baddha - hasta - śīrṣa - āsana
Bound - hand - head - posture
बद्ध - हस्त - शीर्ष - आसन
बद्धहस्तशीर्षासन

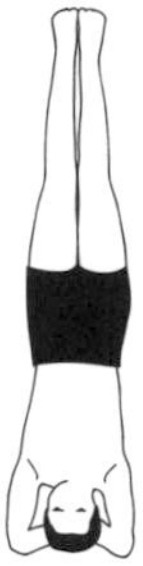

:21 Baddha-Koṇāsana
Baddha - koṇa - āsana
Bound - angle - posture
बद्ध - कोण - आसन
बद्धकोणासन

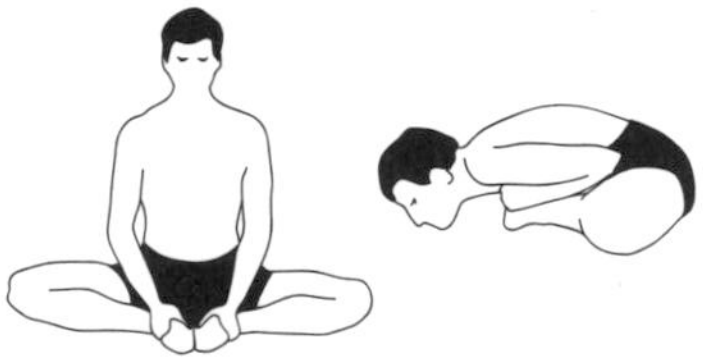

:36 Baddha-Koṇa-Śīrṣāsana
Baddha - koṇa - śīrṣa - āsana
Bound - angle - head - posture
बद्ध - कोण - शीर्ष - आसन
बद्धकोणशीर्षासन

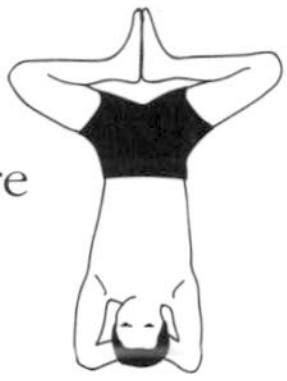

:56 Baddha-Padmāsana
Baddha - padma - āsana
Bound - lotus - posture
बद्ध - पद्म - आसन
बद्धपद्मासन

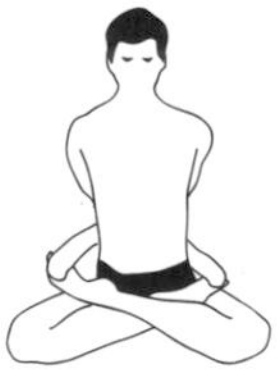

1:10 Bakāsana
Baka - āsana
Crane - posture
बक - आसन
बकासन

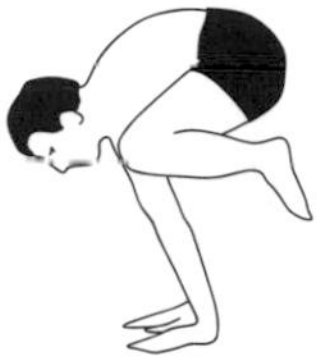

1:20 Bālāsana
Bāla - āsana
Child - posture
बाल - आसन
बालासन

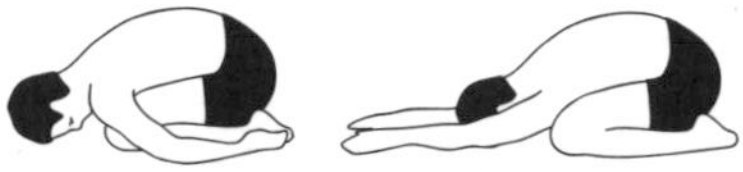

1:32 Bhairavāsana
Bhairava - āsana
Formidable - posture
भैरव - आसन
भैरवासन

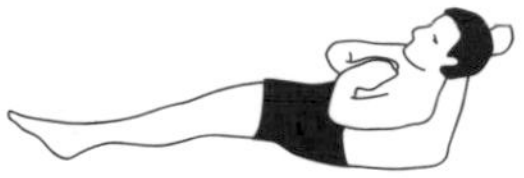

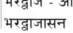

1:45 Bharadvājāsana
Bharadvāja - āsana
(Name of sage) - posture
भरद्वाज - आसन
भरद्वाजासन

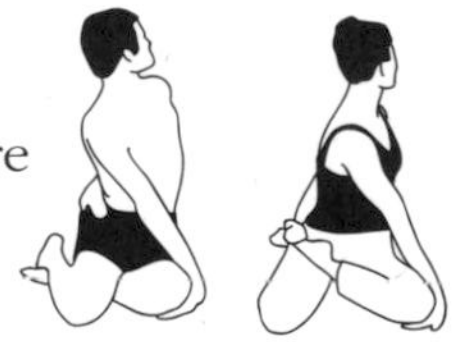

1:59 Bhekāsana
Bheka - āsana
Frog - posture
भेक - आसन
भेकासन

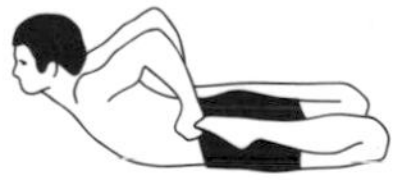

B (continued)

2:10 Bhujaṅgāsana

Bhujaṅga - āsana

Serpent - posture

भुजङ्ग - आसन

भुजङ्गासन

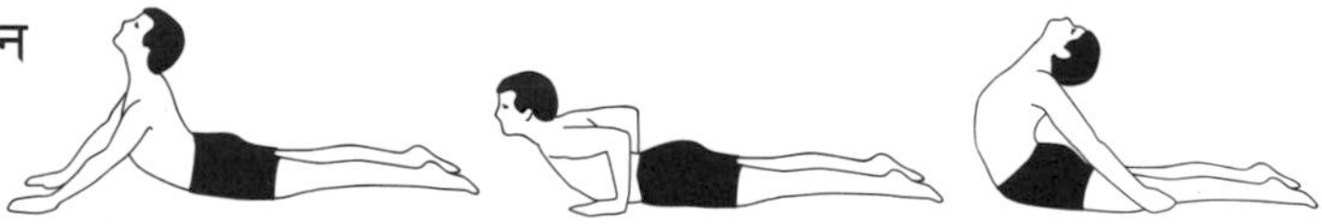

2:23 Bhuja-Pīḍāsana

Bhuja - pīḍa - āsana

Arm - pressure - posture

भुज - पीड - आसन

भुजपीडासन

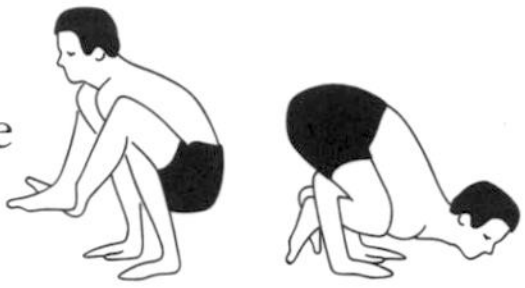

2:39 Buddhāsana

Buddha - āsana

Awakened - posture

बुद्ध - आसन

बुद्धासन

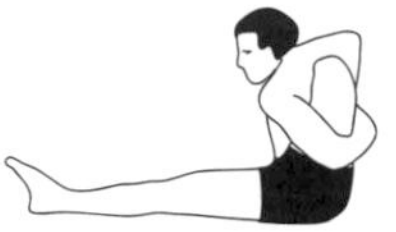

C

DISC 2, TRACK 11
Find individual postures with the time points provided.

:03 Cakorāsana
Cakora - āsana
Partridge - posture
चकोर - आसन
चकोरासन

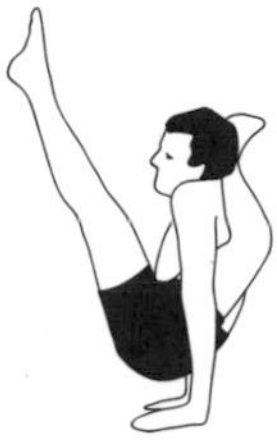

:13 Cakra-Bandhāsana
Cakra - bandha - āsana
Wheel - lock - posture
चक्र - बन्ध - आसन
चक्रबन्धासन

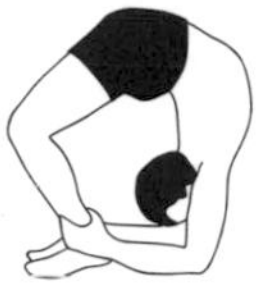

:30 Cakrāsana
Cakra - āsana
Wheel - posture
चक्र - आसन
चक्रासन

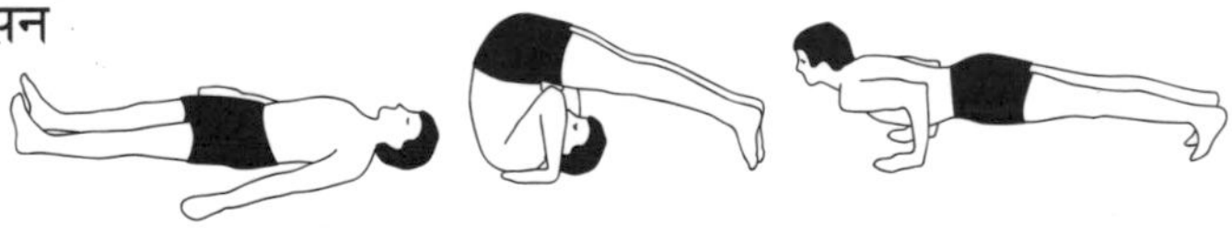

:42 Cakravākāsana
Cakravēka - āsana
Ruddy goose - posture
चक्रवाक - आसन
चक्रवाकासन

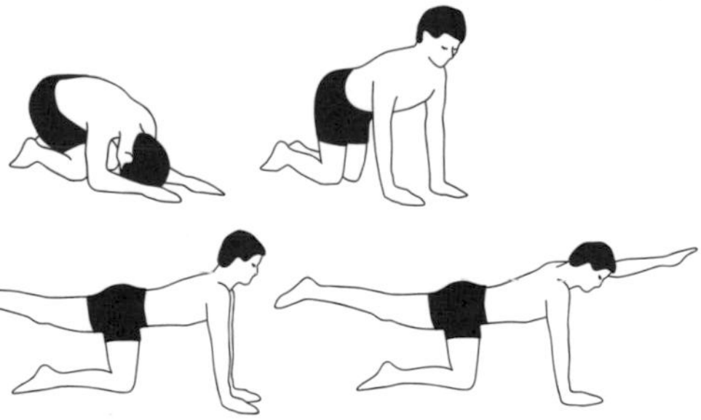

C (continued)

:58 Caturaṅga-Daṇḍāsana

Catur - aṅga - daṇḍa - āsana

Four - limb - staff - posture

चतुर् - अङ्ग - दण्ड - आसन

चतुरङ्गदण्डासन

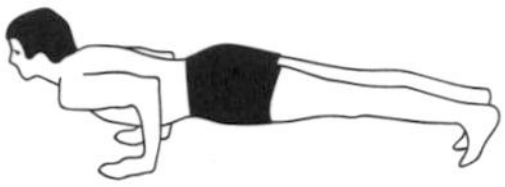

1:16 Catuṣ-Pāda-Pīṭham

Catuṣ - pāda - pīṭham

Four - leg - posture

चतुष् - पाद - पीठम्

चतुष्पादपीठम्

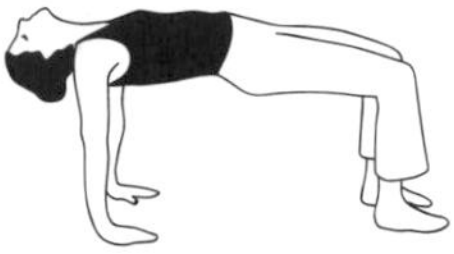

D

DISC 2, TRACK 12
Find individual postures with the time points provided.

:03 Daṇḍāsana
Daṇḍa - āsana
Staff - posture
दण्ड - आसन
दण्डासन

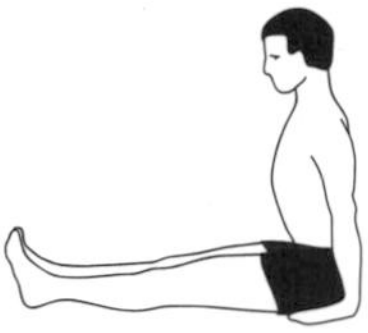

:12 Dhanurāsana
Dhanur - āsana
Bow - posture
धनुर् - आसन
धनुरासन

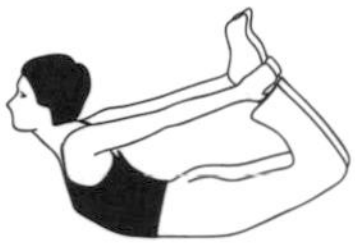

:24 Digāsana
Dig - āsana
Direction - posture
दिग् - आसन
दिगासन

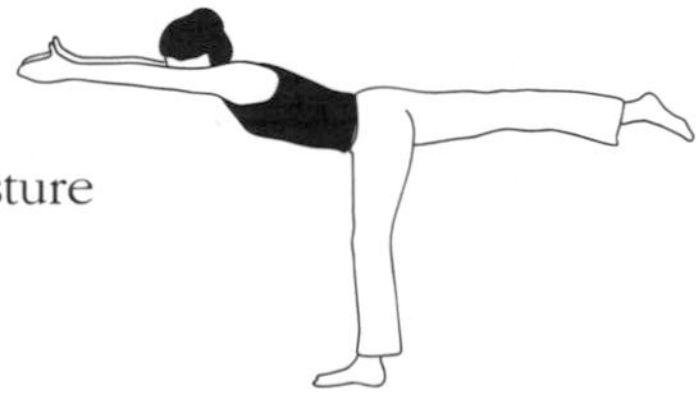

:35 Dūrvāsāsana
Dūrvāsa - āsana
(Name of sage) - posture
दूर्वास - आसन
दूर्वासासन

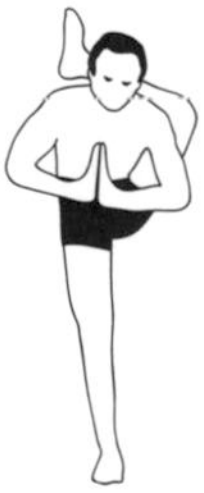

D (continued)

:48 Dvihasta-Bhujāsana
Dvi - hasta - bhuja - āsana
Two - hand - arm - posture
द्वि - हस्त - भुज - आसन
द्विहस्तभुजासन

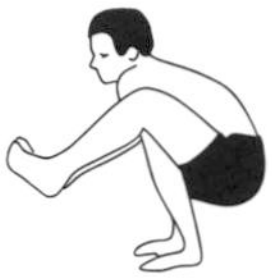

1:07 Dvipāda-Kauṇḍinyāsana
Dvi - pāda - Kauṇḍinya - āsana
Two - leg - (name of sage) - posture
द्वि - पाद् - कौण्डिन्य - आसन
द्विपाद्कौण्डिन्यासन

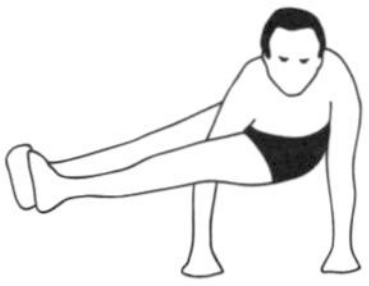

1:29 Dvipāda-Pīṭham
Dvi - pāda - pīṭham
Two - leg - posture
द्वि - पाद् - पीठम्
द्विपाद्पीठम्

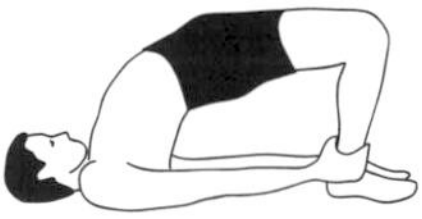

1:46 Dvipāda-Śīrṣāsana
Dvi - pāda - śīrṣa - āsana
Two - leg - head - posture
द्वि - पाद् - शीर्ष - आसन
द्विपाद्शीर्षासन

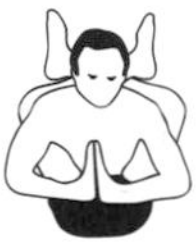

2:05 Dvipāda-Viparīta-Daṇḍāsana
Dvi - pāda - viparīta - daṇḍa - āsana
Two - leg - inverted - staff - posture
द्वि - पाद् - विपरीत - दण्ड - आसन
द्विपाद्विपरीतदण्डासन

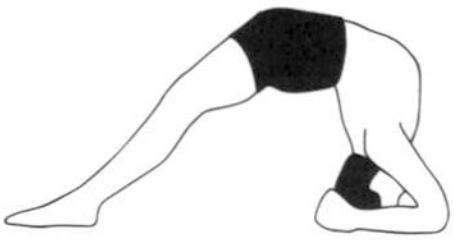

E

DISC 2, TRACK 13
Find individual postures with the time points provided.

:03 Ekahasta-Bhujāsana
Eka - hasta - bhuja - āsana
One - hand - arm - posture
एक - हस्त - भुज - आसन
एकहस्तभुजासन

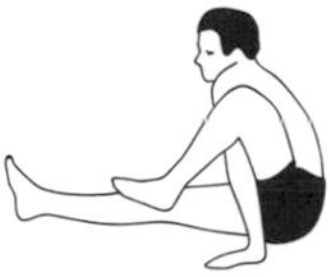

:19 Ekapāda-Bakāsana
Eka - pāda - baka - āsana
One - leg - crane - posture
एक - पाद् - बक - आसन
एकपाद्बकासन

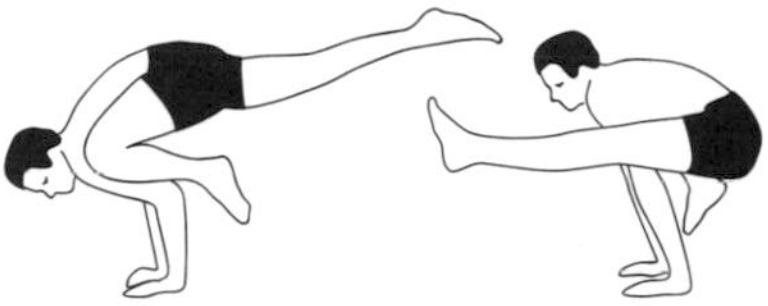

:39 Ekapāda-Gālavāsana
Eka - pāda - Gālava - āsana
One - leg - (name of sage) - posture
एक - पाद् - गालव - आसन
एकपाद्गालवासन

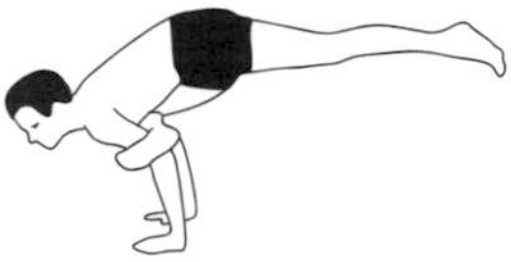

:59 Ekapāda-Kauṇḍinyāsana
Eka - pāda - Kauṇḍinya - āsana
One - leg - (name of sage) - posture
एक - पाद् - कौण्डिन्य - आसन
एकपाद्कौण्डिन्यासन

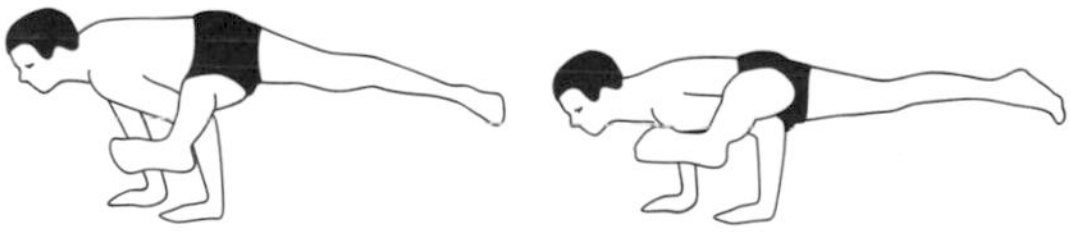

E (continued)

1:21 Ekapāda-Rāja-Kapotāsana

Eka - pāda - rāja - kapota - āsana

One - leg - king - pigeon - posture

एक - पाद् - राज - कपोत - आसन

एकपाद्राजकपोतासन

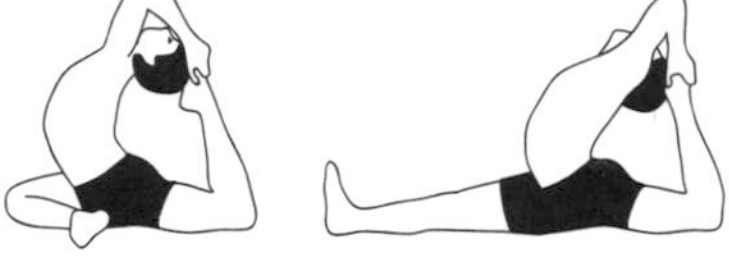

1:44 Ekapāda-Sarvāṅgāsana

Eka - pāda - sarva - aṅga - āsana

One - leg - all - limb - posture

एक - पाद् - सर्व - अङ्ग - आसन

एकपाद्सर्वाङ्गासन

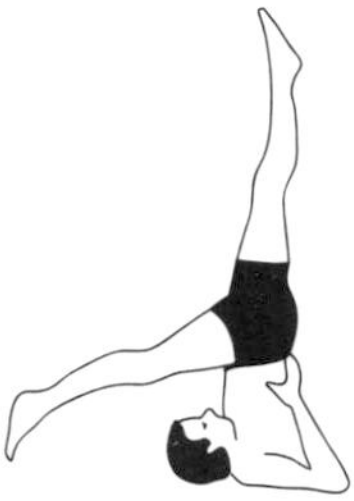

2:09 Ekapāda-Setu-Bandha-Sarvāṅgāsana

Eka - pāda - setu - bandha - sarva - aṅga - āsana

One - leg - bridge - lock - all - limb - posture

एक - पाद् - सेतु - बन्ध - सर्व - अङ्ग - आसन

एकपाद्सेतुबन्धसर्वाङ्गासन

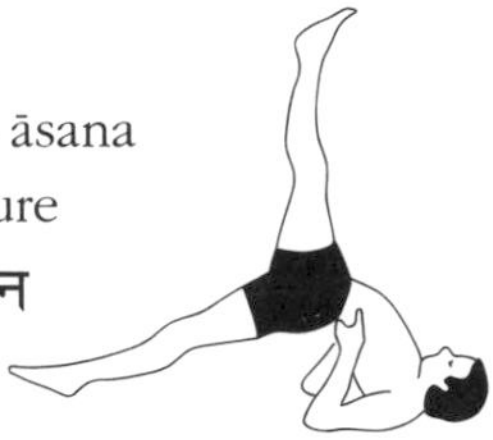

2:40 Ekapāda-Śīrṣāsana

Eka - pāda - śīrṣa - āsana

One - leg - head - posture

एक - पाद् - शीर्ष - आसन

एकपाद्शीर्षासन

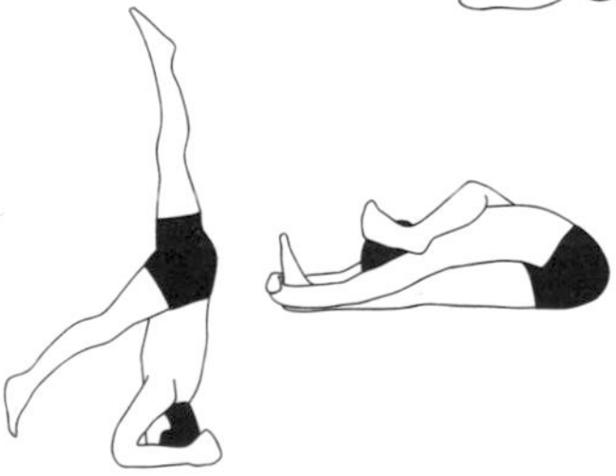

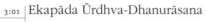

3:01 Ekapāda Ūrdhva-Dhanurāsana

Eka - pāda ūrdhva - dhanur - āsana

One - leg upward - bow - posture

एक - पाद् ऊर्ध्व - धनुर् - आसन

एकपाद् ऊर्ध्वधनुरासन

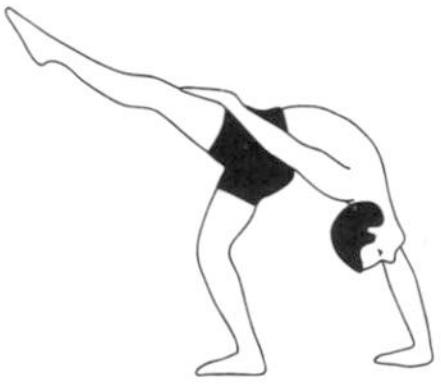

3:25 Ekapāda-Viparīta-Daṇḍāsana

Eka - pāda - viparīta - daṇḍa - āsana

One - leg - inverted - staff - posture

एक - पाद् - विपरीत - दण्ड - आसन

एकपाद्विपरीतदण्डासन

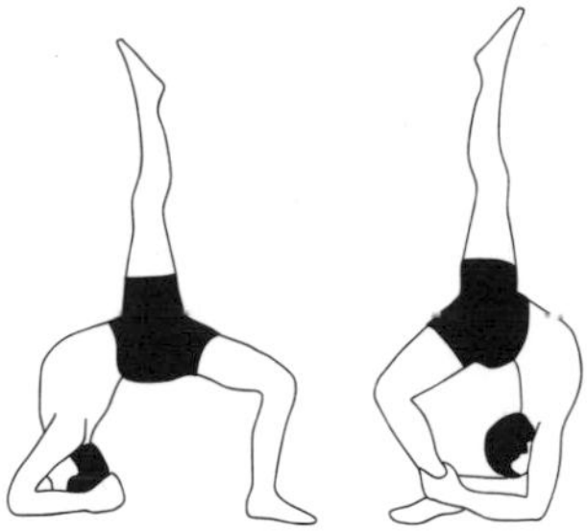

G

DISC 2, TRACK 14
Find individual postures with the time points provided.

:03 Gālavāsana
Gālava - āsana
(Name of sage) - posture
गालव - आसन
गालवासन

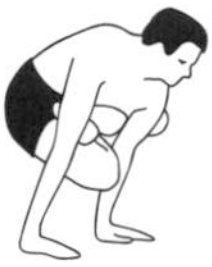

:11 Gaṇḍa-Bheruṇḍāsana
Gaṇḍa - bheruṇḍa - āsana
Side of face - formidable - posture
गण्ड - भेरुण्ड - आसन
गण्डभेरुण्डासन

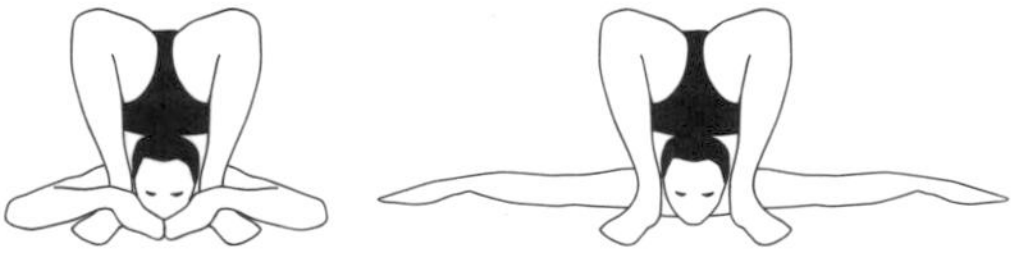

:31 Garbha-Piṇḍāsana
Garbha - piṇḍa - āsana
Womb - ball - posture
गर्भ - पिण्ड - आसन
गर्भपिण्डासन

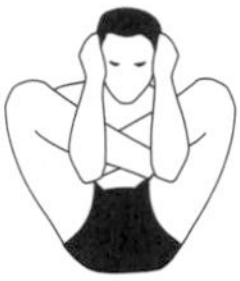

:47 Garuḍāsana
Garuḍa - āsana
Eagle - posture
गरुड - आसन
गरुडासन

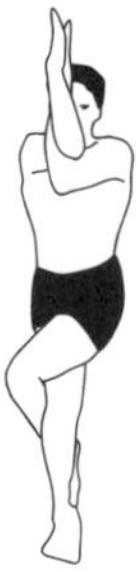

:59 Gheraṇḍāsana
Gheraṇḍa - āsana
(Name of sage) - posture
घेरण्ड - आसन
घेरण्डासन

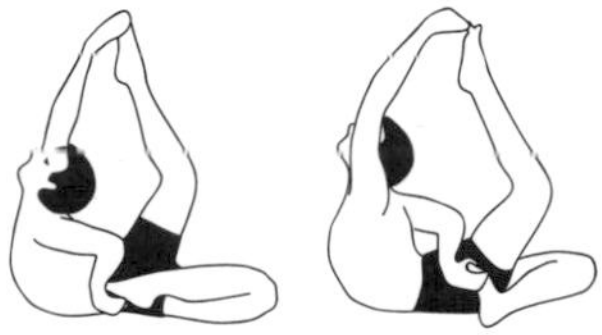

1:11 Godhāpīṭham
Godhā - pīṭham
Alligator - posture
गोधा - पीठम्
गोधापीठम्

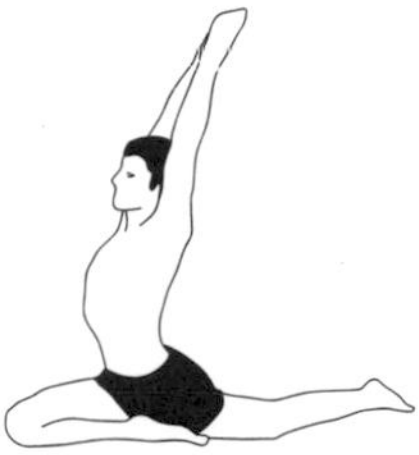

1:25 Go-Mukhāsana
Go - mukha - āsana
Cow - face - posture
गो - मुख - आसन
गोमुखासन

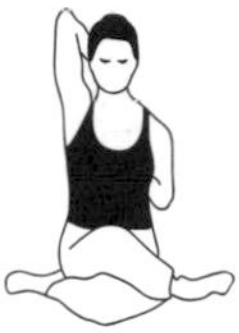

1:39 Gorakṣāsana
Gorakṣa - āsana
Cowherd - posture
गोरक्ष - आसन
गोरक्षासन

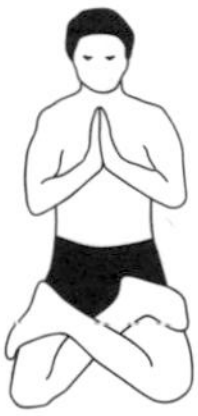

H

DISC 2, TRACK 15
Find individual postures with the time points provided.

:03 Halāsana
Hala - āsana
Plow - posture
हल - आसन
हलासन

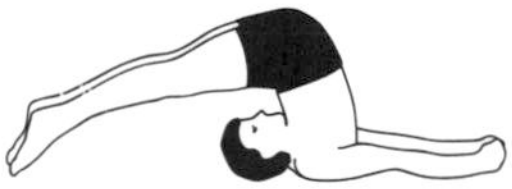

:11 Haṃsāsana
Haṃsa - āsana
Swan - posture
हंस - आसन
हंसासन

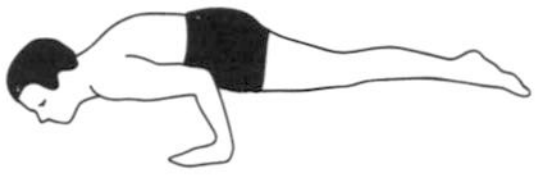

:23 Hanumānāsana
Hanumān - āsana
(Name of monkey deity) - posture
हनुमान् - आसन
हनुमानासन

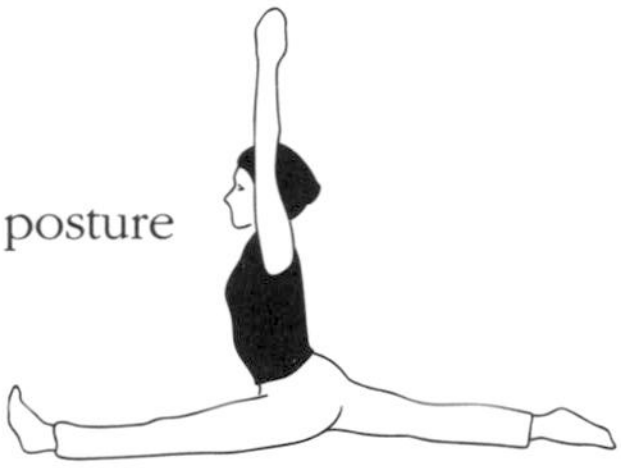

J

DISC 2, TRACK 16
Find individual postures with the time points provided.

:03 Jānu-Śīrṣāsana
Jānu - śīrṣa - āsana
Knee - head - posture
जानु - शीर्ष - आसन
जानुशीर्षासन

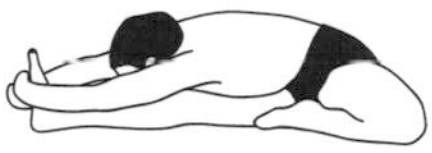

:18 Jaṭhara-Parivartanāsana
Jaṭhara - parivartana - āsana
Stomach - revolving - posture
जठर - परिवर्तन - आसन
जठरपरिवर्तनासन

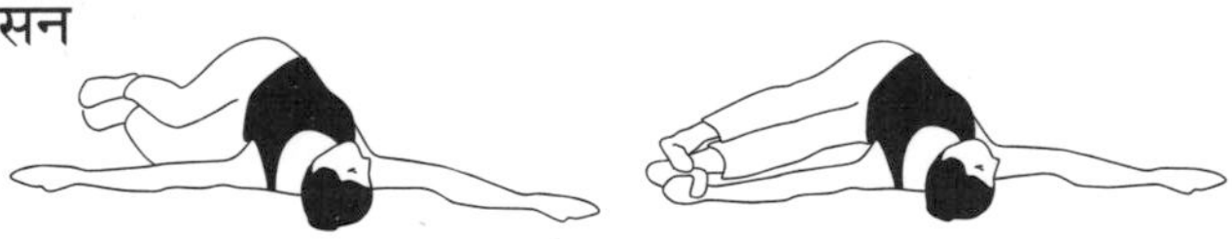

K

DISC 2, TRACK 17
Find individual postures with the time points provided.

:03 Kālabhairavāsana
Kālabhairava - āsana
(Name of Śiva) - posture
कालभैरव - आसन
कालभैरवासन

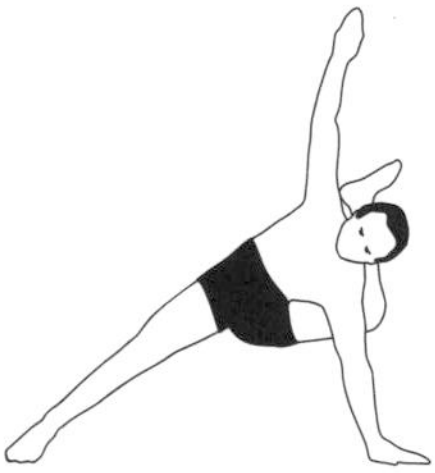

:16 Kandāsana
Kanda - āsana
Knot - posture
कन्द - आसन
कन्दासन

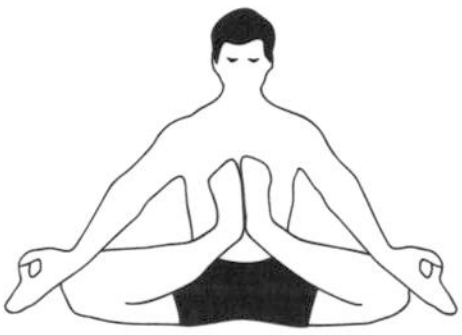

:27 Kapilāsana
Kapila - āsana
(Name of sage) - posture
कपिल - आसन
कपिलासन

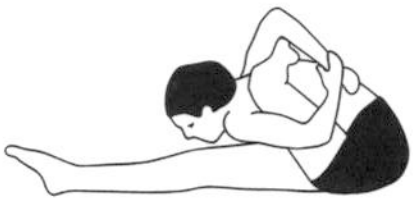

:38 Kapiñjalāsana
Kapiñjala - āsana
Bird that lives on raindrops - posture
कपिञ्जल - आसन
कपिञ्जलासन

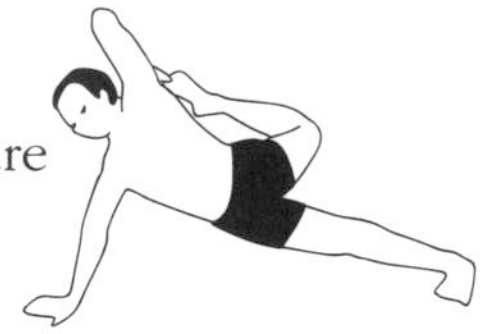

:51 Kapotāsana
Kapota - āsana
Pigeon - posture
कपोत - आसन
कपोतासन

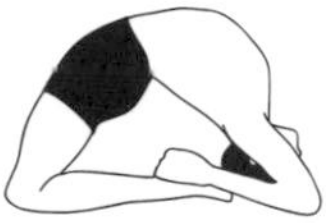

1:03 Kāraṇḍavāsana
Kāraṇḍava - āsana
Himalayan goose - posture
कारण्डव - आसन
कारण्डवासन

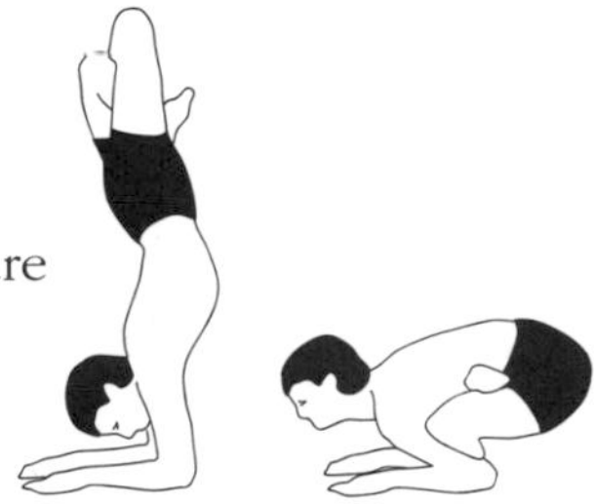

1:18 Karṇapīḍāsana
Karṇa - pīḍa - āsana
Ear - pressure - posture
कर्ण - पीड - आसन
कर्णपीडासन

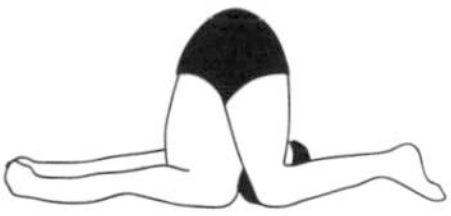

1:34 Kaśyapāsana
Kaśyapa - āsana
(Name of sage) - posture
कश्यप - आसन
कश्यपासन

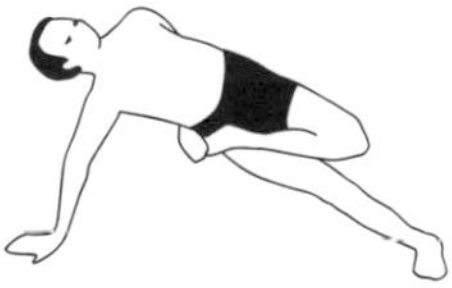

1:45 Krauñcāsana
Krauñca - āsana
Heron - posture
क्रौञ्च - आसन
क्रौञ्चासन

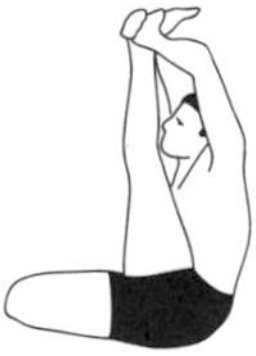

K (continued)

1:51 Kukkuṭāsana
Kukkuṭa - āsana
Rooster - posture
कुक्कुट - आसन
कुक्कुटासन

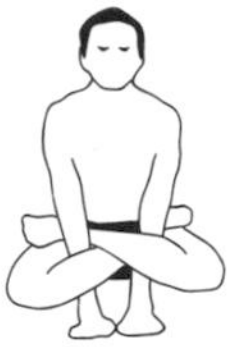

2:09 Kūrmāsana
Kūrma - āsana
Tortoise - posture
कूर्म - आसन
कूर्मासन

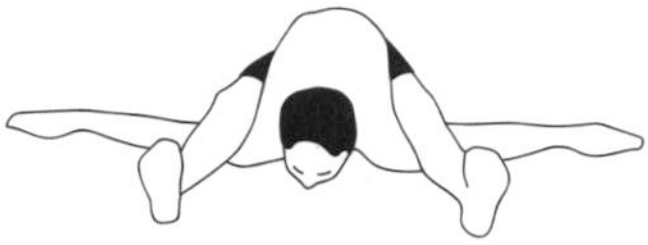

L

DISC 2, TRACK 18
Find individual postures with the time points provided.

:03 Laghu-Vajrāsana
Laghu - vajra - āsana
Light weight - thunderbolt - posture
लघु - वज्र - आसन
लघुवज्रासन

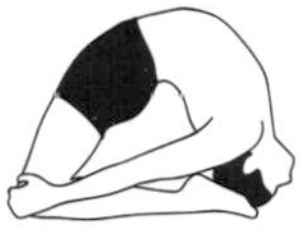

:18 Lolāsana
Lola - āsana
Dangling - posture
लोल - आसन
लोलासन

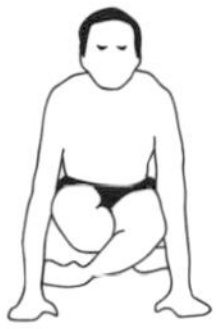

m

DISC 2, TRACK 19
Find individual postures with the time points provided.

:03 | Mahāmudrā
Mahā - mudrā
Great - seal
महा - मुद्रा
महामुद्रा

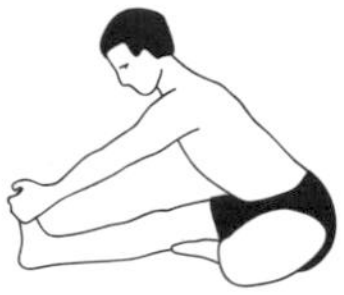

:15 | Makarāsana
Makara - āsana
Sea animal - posture
मकर - आसन
मकरासन

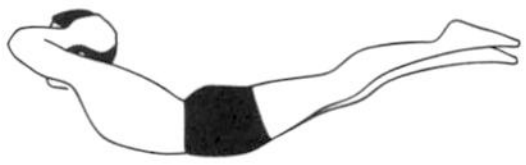

:30 | Mālāsana
Mālā - āsana
Garland - posture
माला - आसन
मालासन

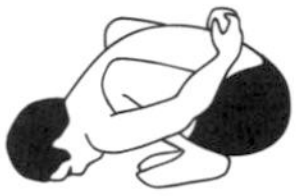

:42 | Maṇḍalāsana
Maṇḍala - āsana
Circle - posture
मण्डल - आसन
मण्डलासन

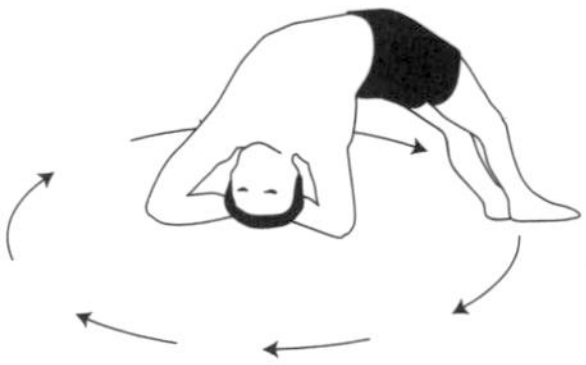

:54 Marīcyāsana
Marīci - āsana
(Name of sage) - posture
मरीचि - आसन
मरीच्यासन

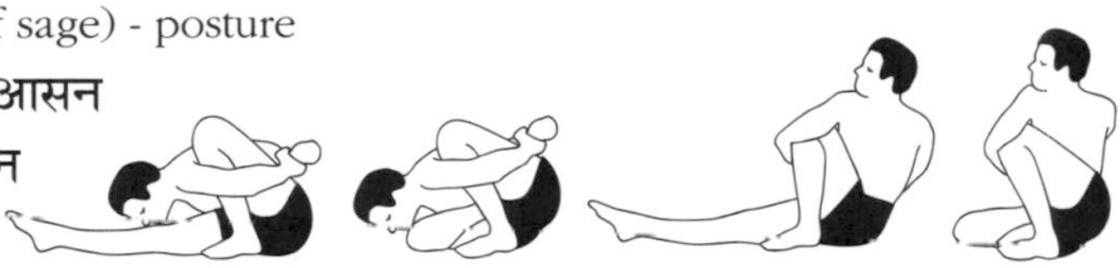

1:06 Matsyāsana
Matsya - āsana
Fish - posture
मत्स्य - आसन
मत्स्यासन

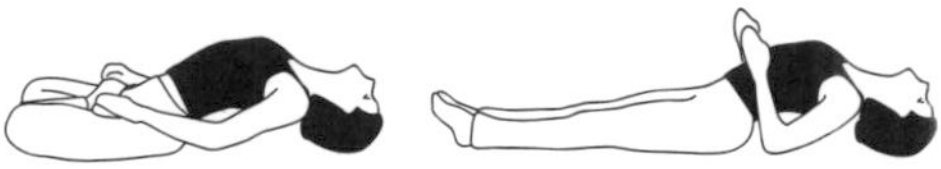

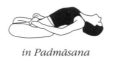

in Padmāsana

1:17 Mayūrāsana
Mayūra - āsana
Peacock - posture
मयूर - आसन
मयूरासन

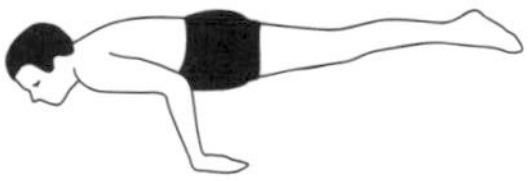

1:29 Mukta-Hasta-Śīrṣāsana
Mukta - hasta - śīrṣa - āsana
Free - hand - head - posture
मुक्त - हस्त - शीर्ष - आसन
मुक्तहस्तशीर्षासन

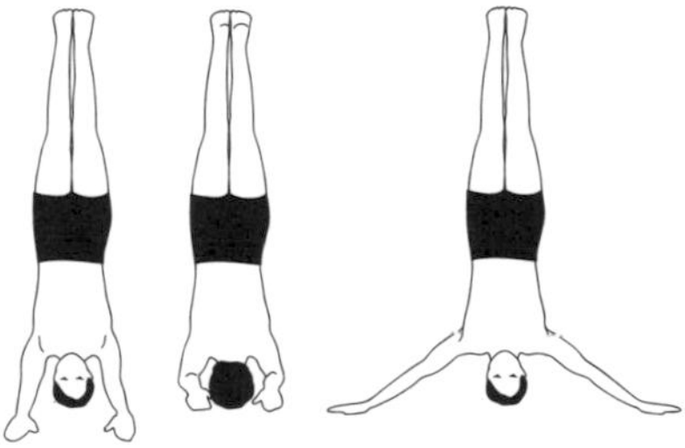

1:49 Mūlabandhāsana
Mūla - bandha - āsana
Root - lock - posture
मूल - बन्ध - आसन
मूलबन्धासन

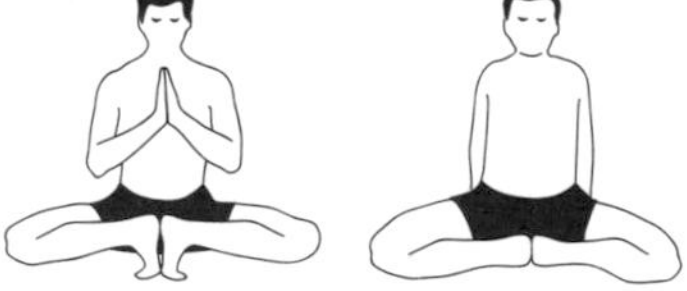

N

DISC 2, TRACK 20
Find individual postures with the time points provided.

:03 Nakrāsana
Nakra - āsana
Crocodile - posture
नक्र - आसन
नक्रासन

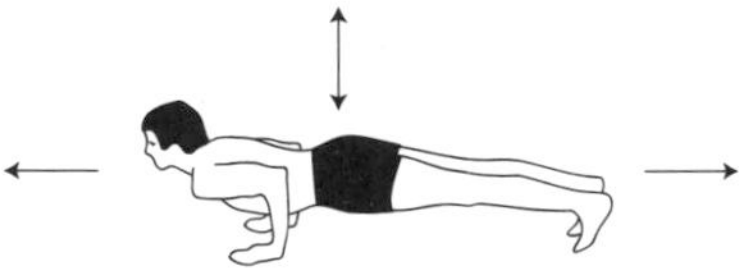

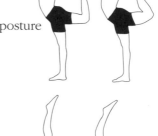

:13 Naṭarājāsana
Naṭarāja - āsana
Lord of the dance (name of Śiva) - posture
नटराज - आसन
नटराजासन

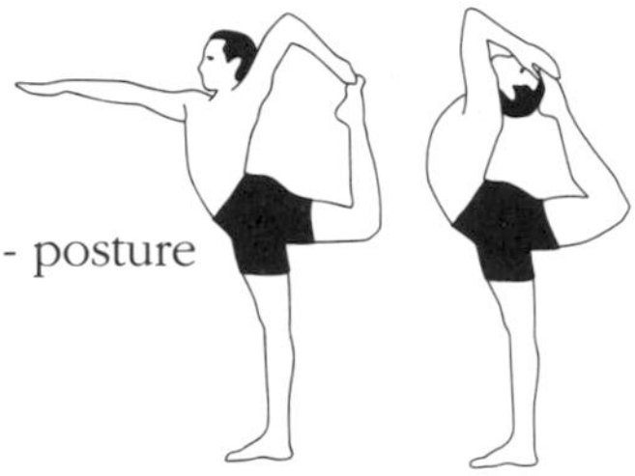

:27 Nirālamba-Sarvāṅgāsana
Nir - ālamba - sarva - aṅga - āsana
Without - support - all - limb - posture
निर् - आलम्ब - सर्व - अङ्ग - आसन
निरालम्बसर्वाङ्गासन

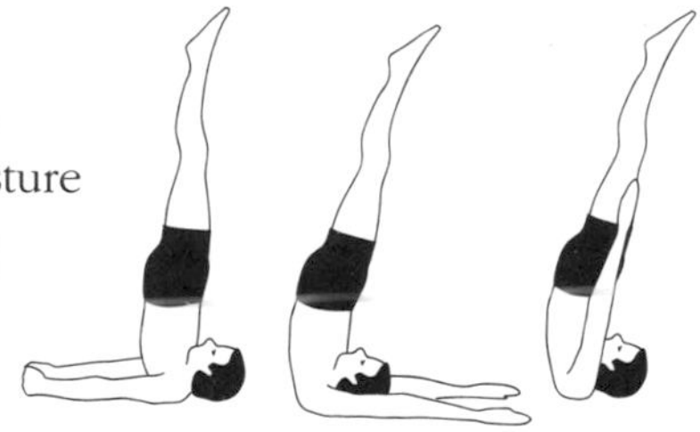

P

DISC 2, TRACK 21
Find individual postures with the time points provided.

:03 Pāda-Hastāsana
Pāda - hasta - āsana
Foot - hand - posture
पाद् - हस्त - आसन
पाद्हस्तासन

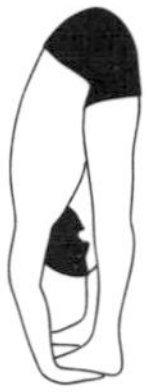

:16 Pādāṅguṣṭha-Dhanurāsana
Pādāṅguṣṭha - dhanur - āsana
Big toe - bow - posture
पादाङ्गुष्ठ - धनुर् - आसन
पादाङ्गुष्ठधनुरासन

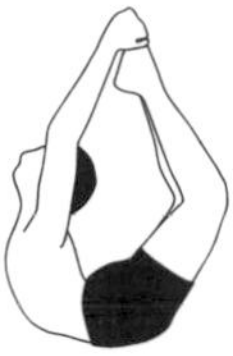

:36 Pādāṅguṣṭhāsana
Pādāṅguṣṭha - āsana
Big toe - posture
पादाङ्गुष्ठ - आसन
पादाङ्गुष्ठासन

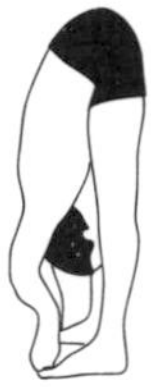

:51 Padma-Mayūrāsana
Padma - mayūra - āsana
Lotus - peacock - posture
पद्म - मयूर - आसन
पद्ममयूरासन

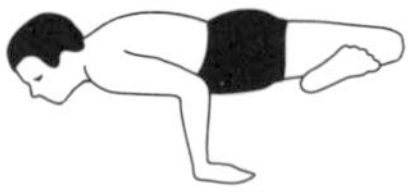

P (continued)

1:07 Padmāsana
Padma - āsana
Lotus - posture
पद्म - आसन
पद्मासन

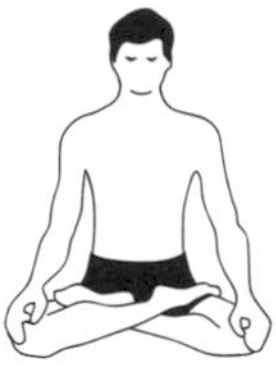

1:17 Parighāsana
Parigha - āsana
Beam (for shutting a gate) - posture
परिघ - आसन
परिघासन

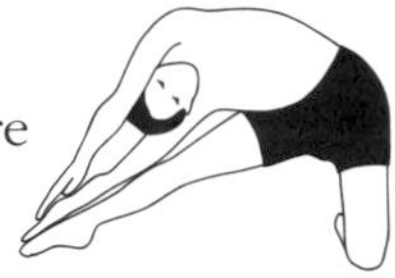

1:30 Paripūrṇa-Matsyendrāsana
Paripūrṇa - matsya - Indra - āsana
Complete - fish - lord - posture
परिपूर्ण - मत्स्य - इन्द्र - आसन
परिपूर्णमत्स्येन्द्रासन

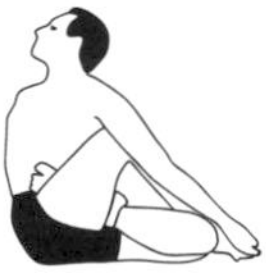

1:51 Paripūrṇa-Nāvāsana
Paripūrṇa - nāva - āsana
Full - boat - posture
परिपूर्ण - नाव - आसन
परिपूर्णनावासन

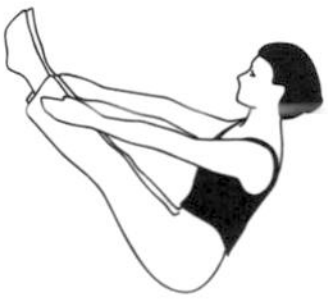

2:08 Parivṛtta-Ardha-Candrāsana
Parivṛtta - ardha - candra - āsana
Revolved - half - moon - posture
परिवृत्त अर्ध - चन्द्र - आसन
परिवृत्त अर्धचन्द्रासन

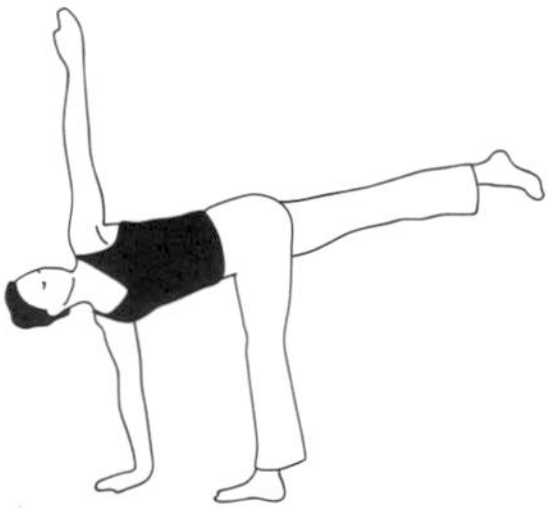

2:30 Parivṛttaikapāda-Śīrṣāsana

Parivṛtta - eka - pāda - śīrṣa - āsana

Revolved - one - leg - head - posture

परिवृत्त - एक - पाद् - शीर्ष - आसन

परिवृत्तैकपाद्शीर्षासन

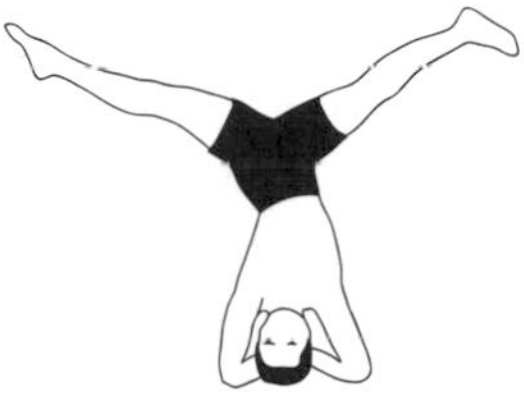

2:54 Parivṛtta-Jānu-Śīrṣāsana

Parivṛtta - jānu - śīrṣa - āsana

Revolved - knee - head - posture

परिवृत्त - जानु - शीर्ष - आसन

परिवृत्तजानुशीर्षासन

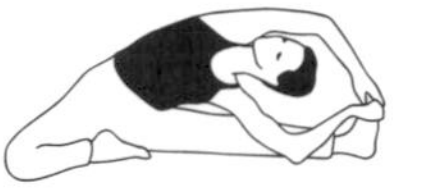

3:16 Parivṛtta-Pārśvakoṇāsana

Parivṛtta - pārśva - koṇa - āsana

Revolved - side - angle - posture

परिवृत्त - पार्श्व - कोण - आसन

परिवृत्तपार्श्वकोणासन

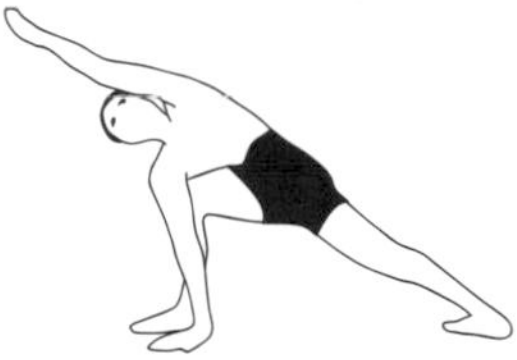

3:36 Parivṛtta-Paścimottānāsana

Parivṛtta - paścima - uttāna - āsana

Revolved - back - stretched out - posture

परिवृत्त - पश्चिम - उत्तान - आसन

परिवृत्तपश्चिमोत्तानासन

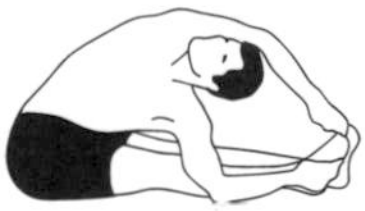

3:58 Parivṛtta-Trikoṇāsana

Parivṛtta - trikoṇa - āsana

Revolved - triangle - posture

परिवृत्त - त्रिकोण - आसन

परिवृत्तत्रिकोणासन

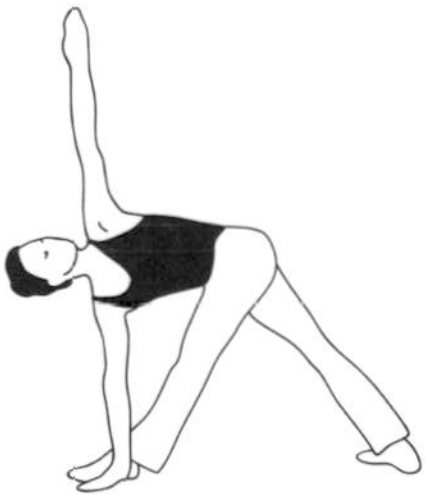

P (continued)

4:16 Pārśva-Bakāsana
Pārśva - baka - āsana
Side - crane - posture
पार्श्व - बक - आसन
पार्श्वबकासन

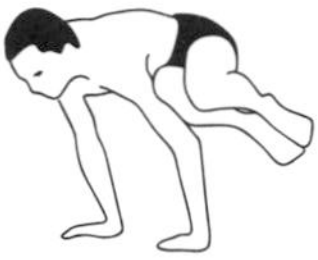

4:31 Pārśva-Dhanurāsana
Pārśva - dhanur - āsana
Side - bow - posture
पार्श्व - धनुर् - आसन
पार्श्वधनुरासन

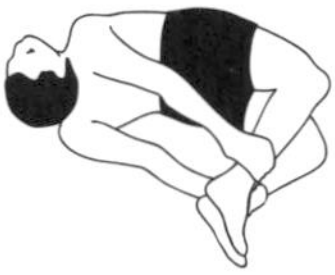

4:47 Pārśva-Halāsana
Pārśva - hala - āsana
Side - plow - posture
पार्श्व - हल - आसन
पार्श्वहलासन

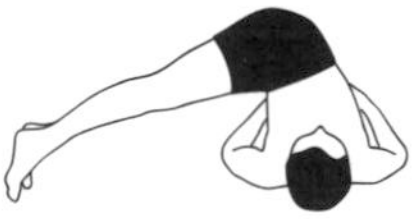

5:02 Pārśva-Kukkuṭāsana
Pārśva - kukkuṭa - āsana
Side - rooster - posture
पार्श्व - कुक्कुट - आसन
पार्श्वकुक्कुटासन

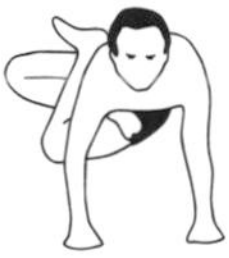

5:18 Pārśva-Piṇḍāsana
Pārśva - piṇḍa - āsana
Side - ball - posture
पार्श्व - पिण्ड - आसन
पार्श्वपिण्डासन

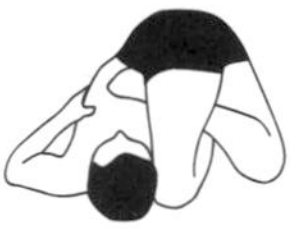

5:33 Pārśva-Sarvāṅgāsana

Pārśva - sarva - aṅga - āsana

Side - all - limb - posture

पार्श्व - सर्व - अङ्ग - आसन

पार्श्वसर्वाङ्गासन

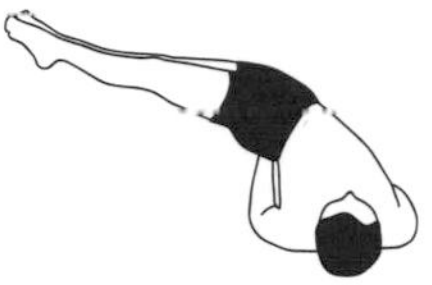

5:53 Pārśva-Śīrṣāsana

Pārśva - śīrṣa - āsana

Side - head - posture

पार्श्व - शीर्ष - आसन

पार्श्वशीर्षासन

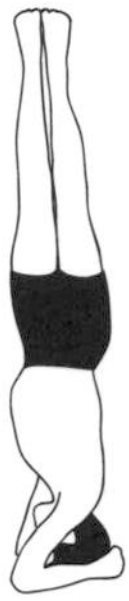

6:11 Pārśva-Upaviṣṭa-Koṇāsana

Pārśva upaviṣṭa- koṇa - āsana

Side seated - angle - posture

पार्श्व उपविष्ट - कोण - आसन

पार्श्व उपविष्टकोणासन

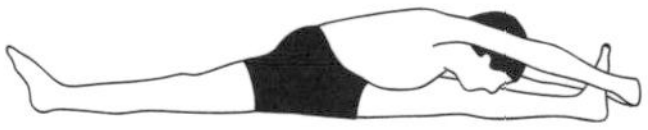

6:32 Pārśva-Ūrdhva-Padmāsana

Pārśva ūrdhva - padma - āsana

Side upward - lotus - posture

पार्श्व ऊर्ध्व - पद्म - आसन

पार्श्व ऊर्ध्वपद्मासन

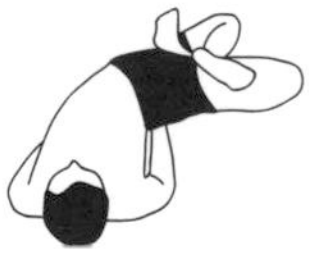

in Sarvāṅgāsana

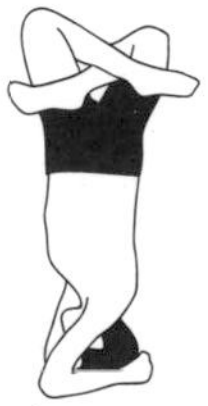

in Śīrṣāsana

6:51 Pārśvaikapāda-Sarvāṅgāsana

Pārśva - eka - pāda - sarva - aṅga - āsana

Side - one - leg - all - limb - posture

पार्श्व - एक - पाद - सर्व - अङ्ग - आसन

पार्श्वैकपादसर्वाङ्गासन

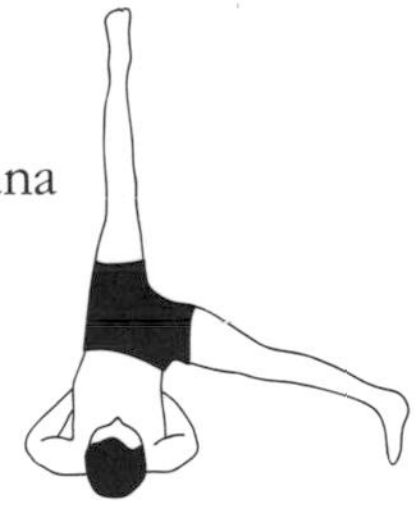

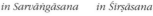

P (continued)

7:19 Pārśvaikapāda-Śīrṣāsana
Pārśva - eka - pāda - śīrṣa - āsana
Side - one - leg - head - posture
पार्श्व - एक - पाद् - शीर्ष - आसन
पार्श्वैकपादशीर्षासन

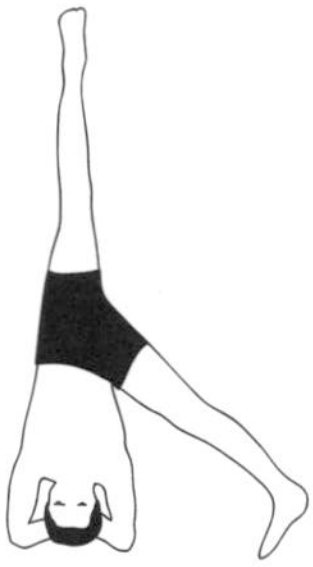

7:43 Pārśvottānāsana
Pārśva - uttāna - āsana
Side - stretched out - posture
पार्श्व - उत्तान - आसन
पार्श्वोत्तानासन

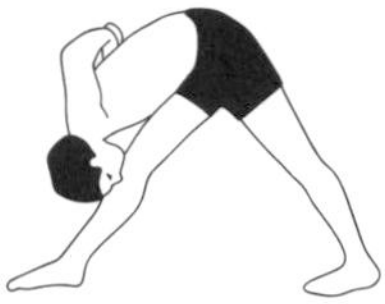

7:59 Parvatāsana
Parvata - āsana
Mountain - posture
पर्वत - आसन
पर्वतासन

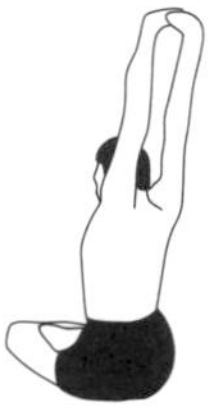

8:10 Paryaṅkāsana
Paryaṅka - āsana
Couch - posture
पर्यङ्क - आसन
पर्यङ्कासन

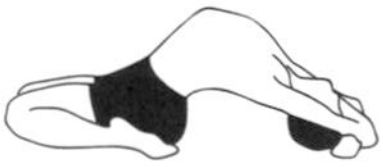

8:22 Pāśāsana
Pāśa - āsana
Noose - posture
पाश - आसन
पाशासन

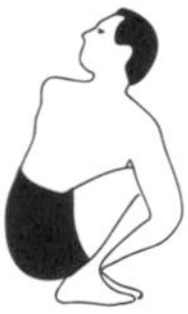

8:32 Paścimottānāsana

Paścima - uttāna - āsana

Back - stretched out - posture

पश्चिम - उत्तान - आसन

पश्चिमोत्तानासन

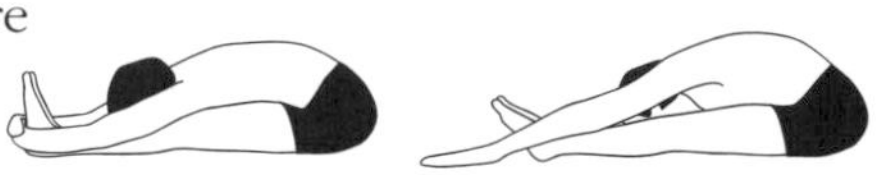

8:49 Pīñca-Mayūrāsana

Pīñca - mayūra - āsana

Feather - peacock - posture

पीञ्च - मयूर - आसन

पीञ्चमयूरासन

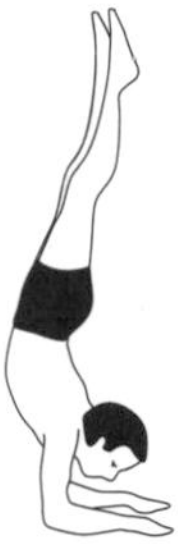

9:08 Piṇḍāsana

Piṇḍa - āsana

Ball - posture

पिण्ड - आसन

पिण्डासन

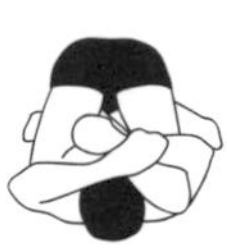

in Sarvāṅgāsana

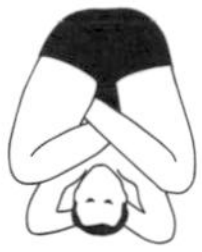

in Śīrṣāsana

9:19 Prasārita Pādottānāsana

Prasārita pāda - uttāna - āsana

Spread leg - stretched out - posture

प्रसारित पाद् - उत्तान - आसन

प्रसारितपादोत्तानासन

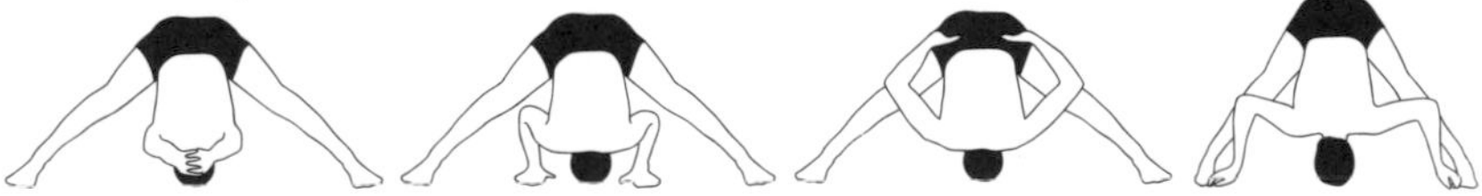

9:40 Pūrvottānāsana

Pūrva - uttāna - āsana

Front - stretched out - posture

पूर्व - उत्तान - आसन

पूर्वोत्तानासन

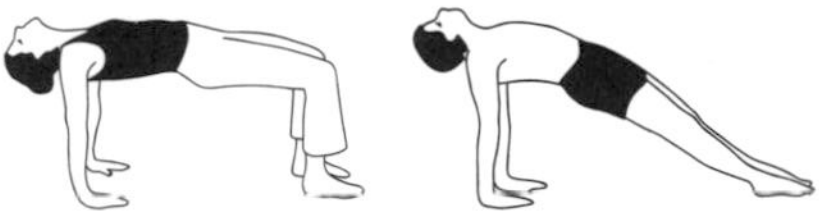

R

DISC 2, TRACK 22
Find individual postures with the time points provided.

:03 Rāja-Kapotāsana
Rāja - kapota - āsana
King - pigeon - posture
राज - कपोत - आसन
राजकपोतासन

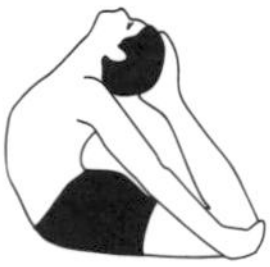

:18 Ṛcīkāsana
Ṛcīka - āsana
(Name of sage) - posture
ऋचीक - आसन
ऋचीकासन

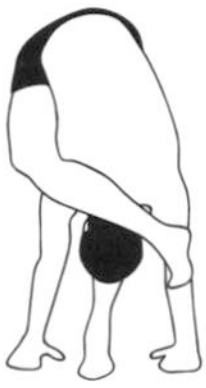

S

DISC 2, TRACK 23
Find individual postures with the time points provided.

:03 Śalabhāsana
Śalabha - āsana
Locust - posture
शलभ - आसन
शलभासन

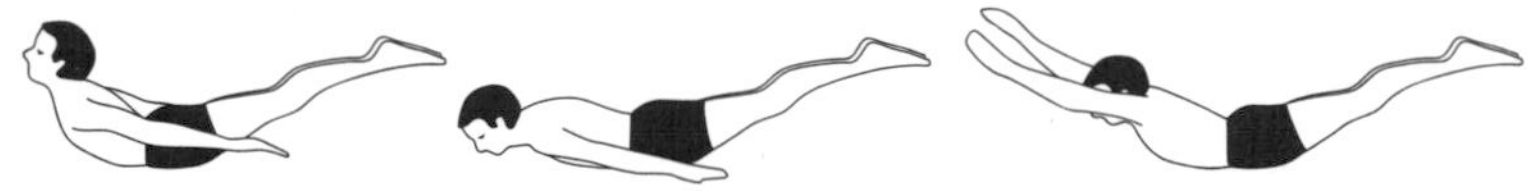

:14 Sālamba-Sarvāṅgāsana
Sa - ālamba - sarva - aṅga - āsana
With - support - all - limb - posture
स - आलम्ब - सर्व - अङ्ग - आसन
सालम्बसर्वाङ्गासन

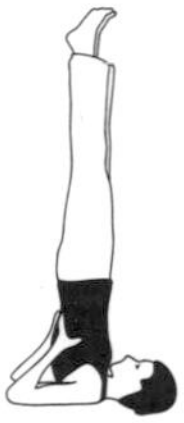

:40 Sālamba-Śīrṣāsana
Sa - ālamba - śīrṣa - āsana
With - support - head - posture
स - आलम्ब - शीर्ष - आसन
सालम्बशीर्षासन

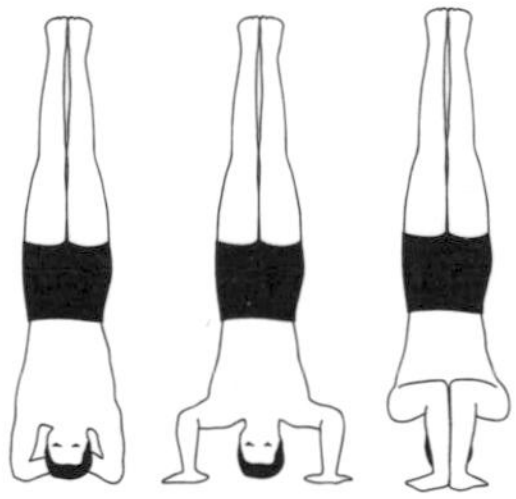

1:00 Samakoṇāsana
Sama - koṇa - āsana
Equal - angle - posture
सम - कोण - आसन
समकोणासन

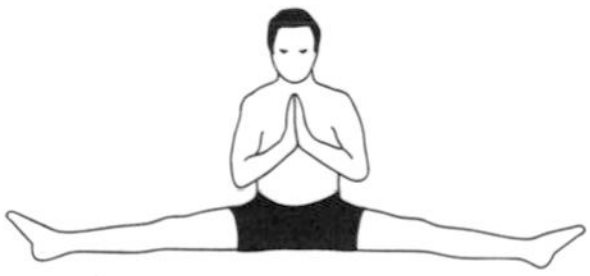

S (continued)

1:14 Samasthiti
Sama - sthiti
Equal - standing
सम - स्थिति
समस्थिति

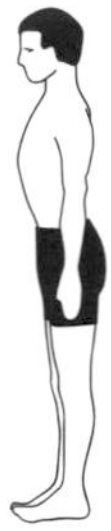

1:28 Ṣanmukhī-Mudrā
Ṣan - mukhī - mudrā
Six - faced - seal
षन् - मुखी - मुद्रा
षन्मुखीमुद्रा

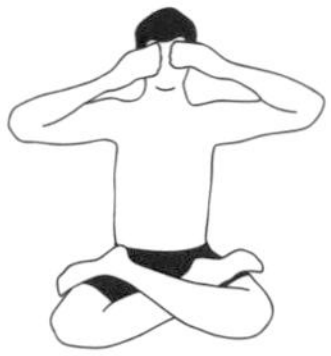

1:48 Śavāsana
Śava - āsana
Corpse - posture
शव - आसन
शवासन

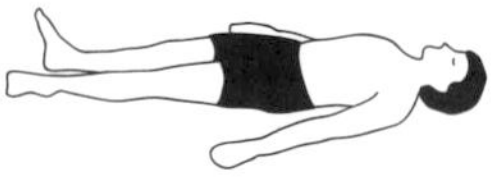

1:59 Śayanāsana
Śayana - āsana
Relaxing - posture
शयन - आसन
शयनासन

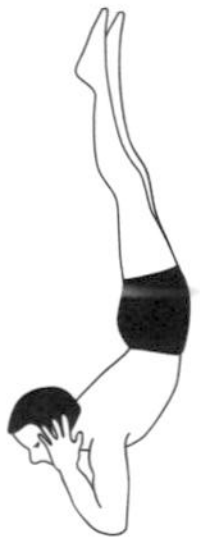

2:11 Setubandha-Sarvāṅgāsana
Setu - bandha - sarva - aṅga - āsana
Bridge - lock - all - limb - posture
सेतु - बन्ध - सर्व - अङ्ग - आसन
सेतुबन्धसर्वाङ्गासन

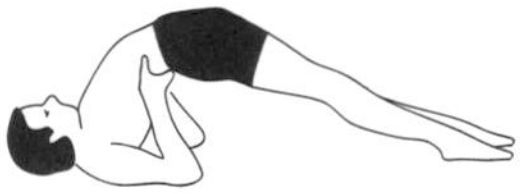

2:35 Setu-Bandhāsana
Setu - bandha - āsana
Bridge - lock - posture
सेतु - बन्ध - आसन
सेतुबन्धासन

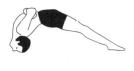

2:51 Siddhāsana
Siddha - āsana
Accomplished - posture
सिद्ध - आसन
सिद्धासन

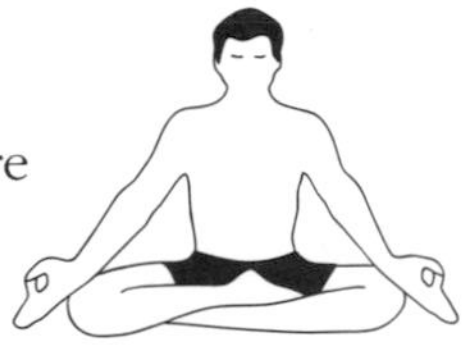

3:03 Siṃhāsana
Siṃha - āsana
Lion - posture
सिंह - आसन
सिंहासन

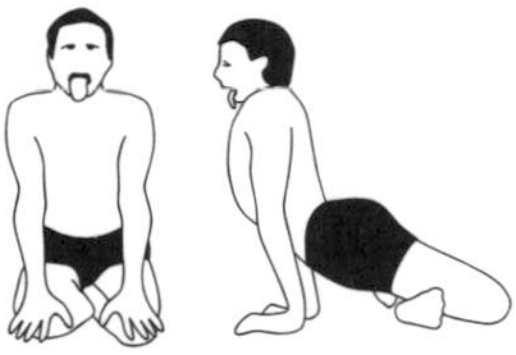

3:14 Śīrṣa-Pādāsana
Śīrṣa - pāda - āsana
Head - foot - posture
शीर्ष - पाद - आसन
शीर्षपादासन

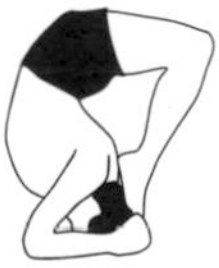

3:31 Skandāsana
Skanda - āsana
(Name of sage) - posture
स्कन्द - आसन
स्कन्दासन

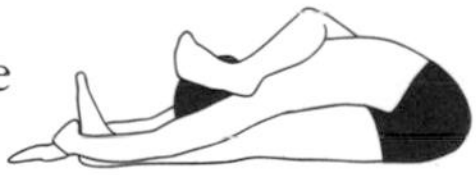

S (continued)

3:41 Sukhāsana
Sukha - āsana
Easy - posture
सुख - आसन
सुखासन

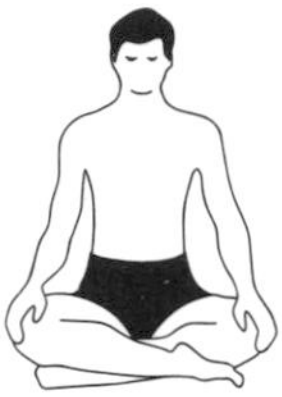

3:52 Supta-Baddha-Koṇāsana
Supta - baddha - koṇa - āsana
Supine - bound - angle - posture
सुप्त - बद्ध - कोण - आसन
सुप्तबद्धकोणासन

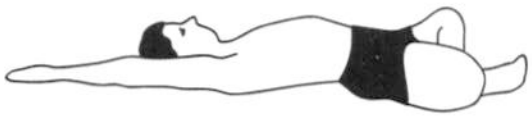

4:12 Supta-Bhekāsana
Supta - bheka - āsana
Supine - frog - posture
सुप्त - भेक - आसन
सुप्तभेकासन

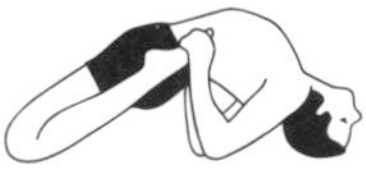

4:27 Supta-Daṇḍāsana
Supta - daṇḍa - āsana
Supine - staff - posture
सुप्त - दण्ड - आसन
सुप्तदण्डासन

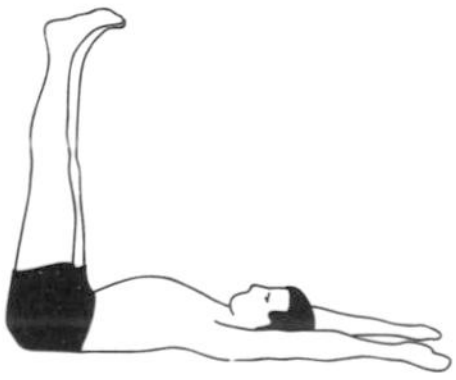

4:42 Supta-Koṇāsana
Supta - koṇa - āsana
Supine - angle - posture
सुप्त - कोण - आसन
सुप्तकोणासन

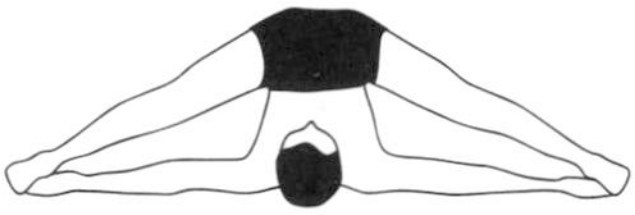

4:56 Supta-Kūrmāsana
Supta - kūrma - āsana
Supine - tortoise - posture
सुप्त - कूर्म - आसन
सुप्तकूर्मासन

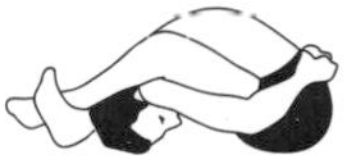

5:11 Supta-Pādāṅguṣṭhāsana
Supta - pādāṅguṣṭha - āsana
Supine - big toe - posture
सुप्त - पादाङ्गुष्ठ - आसन
सुप्तपादाङ्गुष्ठासन

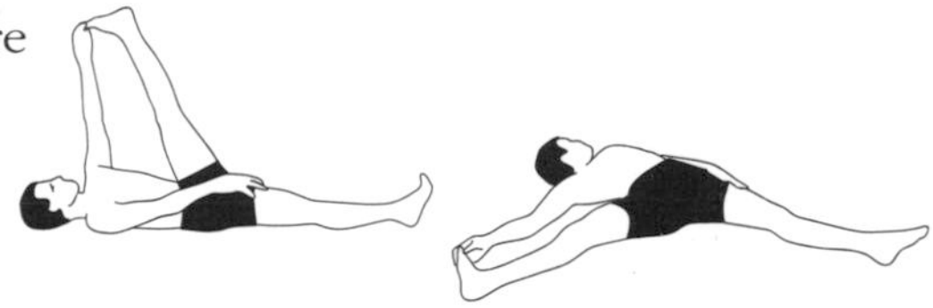

5:29 Supta-Trivikramāsana
Supta - tri - vikrama - āsana
Supine - three - stride - posture
सुप्त - त्रि - विक्रम - आसन
सुप्तत्रिविक्रमासन

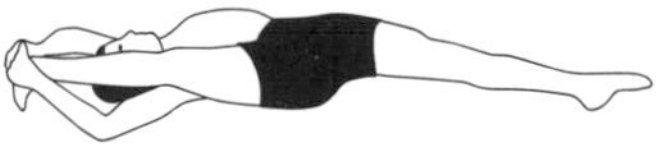

5:49 Supta-Ūrdhva-Pāda-Vajrāsana
Supta ūrdhva - pāda - vajra - āsana
Supine upwards - foot - thunderbolt - posture
सुप्त ऊर्ध्व - पाद - वज्र - आसन
सुप्त ऊर्ध्वपादवज्रासन

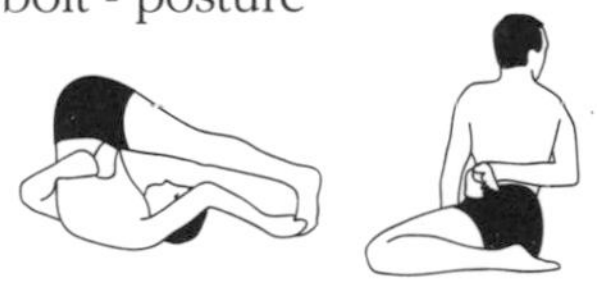

6:13 Supta-Vajrāsana
Supta - vajra - āsana
Supine - thunderbolt - posture
सुप्त - वज्र - आसन
सुप्तवज्रासन

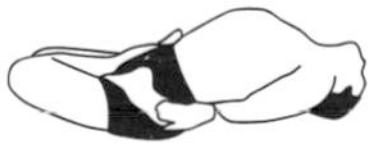

S (continued)

6:28 Supta-Vīrāsana
Supta - vīra - āsana
Supine - hero - posture
सुप्त - वीर - आसन
सुप्तवीरासन

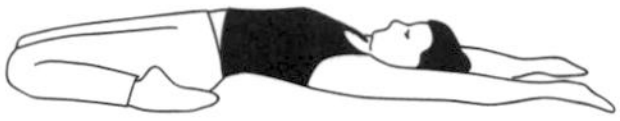

6:43 Sūrya-Namaskāra
Sūrya - namaskāra
Sun - salutation
सूर्य - नमस्कार
सूर्यनमस्कार

A series of postures with numerous variations, one of which is in the Aṣṭāṅga section

6:58 Svastikāsana
Svastika - āsana
Auspicious - posture
स्वस्तिक - आसन
स्वस्तिकासन

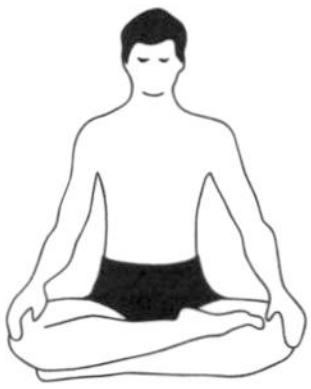

T

DISC 2, TRACK 24
Find individual postures with the time points provided.

:03 Taḍāka-Mudrā
Taḍāka - mudrā
Pond gesturc
तडाक - मुद्रा
तडाकमुद्रा

:17 Tāḍāsana
Tāḍa - āsana
Mountain - posture
ताड - आसन
ताडासन

:28 Tiryaṅ-Mukhaikapāda-Paścimottānāsana
Tiryaṅ - mukha - eka - pāda - paścima - uttāna - āsana
Oblique - face - one - leg - back - stretched out - posture
तिर्यङ् - मुख - एक - पाद - पश्चिम - उत्तान - आसन
तिर्यङ्मुखैकपादपश्चिमोत्तानासन

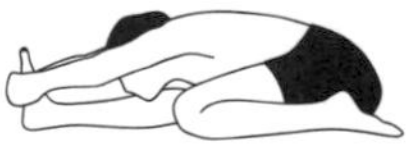

1:03 Tiryaṅ-Mukhottānāsana
Tiryaṅ - mukha - uttāna - āsana
Upside down - face - stretched out - posture
तिर्यङ् - मुख - उत्तान - आसन
तिर्यङ्मुखोत्तानासन

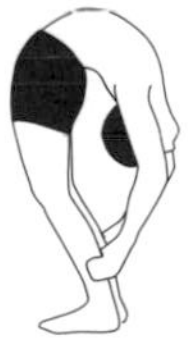

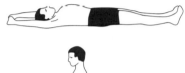

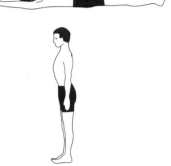

T (continued)

1:28 Tittibhāsana
Tittibha - āsana
Firefly - posture
तित्तिभ - आसन
तित्तिभासन

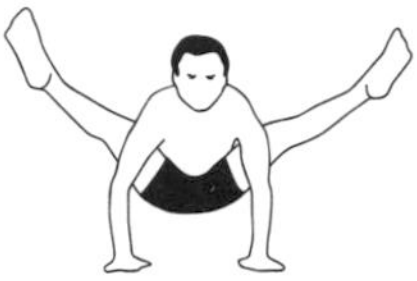

1:40 Tolāsana
Tola - āsana
Scale (for weighing) - posture
तोल - आसन
तोलासन

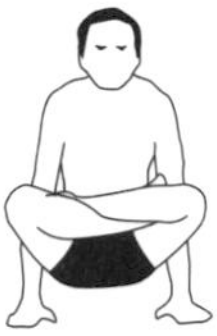

1:50 Trivikramāsana
Tri - vikrama - āsana
Three - stride - posture
त्रि - विक्रम - आसन
त्रिविक्रमासन

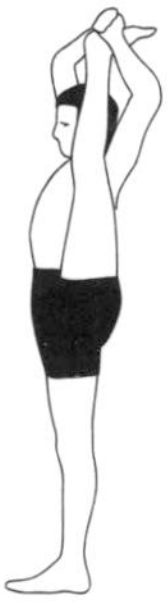

U

DISC 2, TRACK 25
Find individual postures with the time points provided.

:03 Ubhaya-Pādāṅguṣṭhāsana
Ubhaya - pādāṅguṣṭha - āsana
Both - big toe - posture
उभय - पादाङ्गुष्ठ - आसन
उभयपादाङ्गुष्ठासन

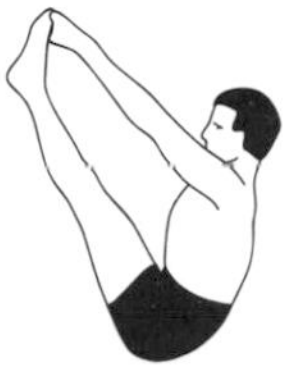

:21 Upaviṣṭa-Koṇāsana
Upaviṣṭa - koṇa - āsana
Seated - angle - posture
उपविष्ट - कोण - आसन
उपविष्टकोणासन

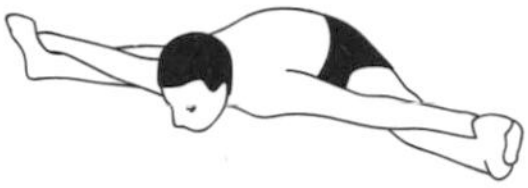

:37 Ūrdhva-Daṇḍāsana
Ūrdhva - daṇḍa - āsana
Upward - staff - posture
ऊर्ध्व - दण्ड - आसन
ऊर्ध्वदण्डासन

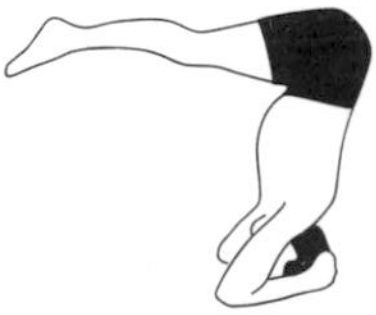

:53 Ūrdhva-Dhanurāsana
Ūrdhva - dhanur - āsana
Upward - bow - posture
ऊर्ध्व - धनुर् - आसन
ऊर्ध्वधनुरासन

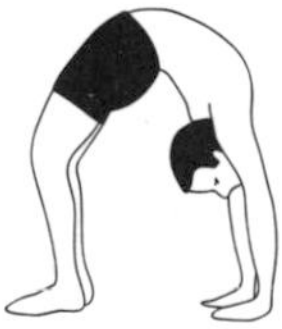

U (continued)

1:09 Ūrdhva-Kukkuṭāsana
Ūrdhva - kukkuṭa - āsana
Upward - rooster - posture
ऊर्ध्व - कुक्कुट - आसन
ऊर्ध्वकुक्कुटासन

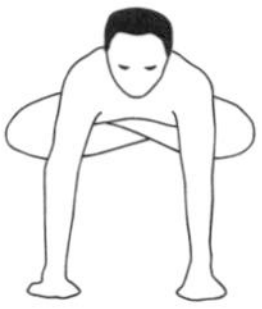

1:25 Ūrdhva-Mukha-Paścimottānāsana
Ūrdhva - mukha - paścima - uttāna - āsana
Upward - facing - back - stretched out - posture
ऊर्ध्व - मुख - पश्चिम - उत्तान - आसन
ऊर्ध्वमुखपश्चिमोत्तानासन

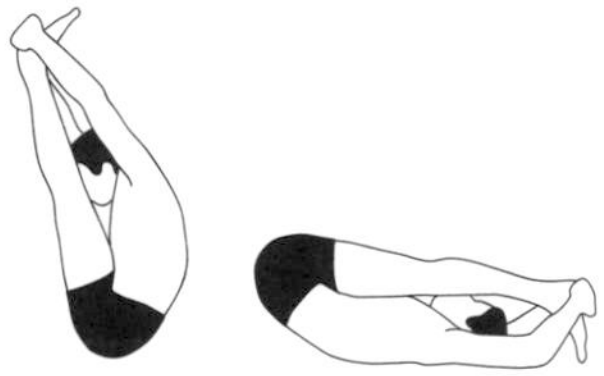

1:53 Ūrdhva-Mukha-Śvānāsana
Ūrdhva - mukha - śvāna - āsana
Upward - facing - dog - posture
ऊर्ध्व - मुख - श्वान - आसन
ऊर्ध्वमुखश्वानासन

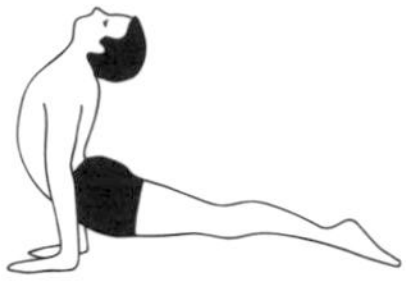

2:12 Ūrdhva-Padmāsana
Ūrdhva - padma - āsana
Upward - lotus - posture
ऊर्ध्व - पद्म - आसन
ऊर्ध्वपद्मासन

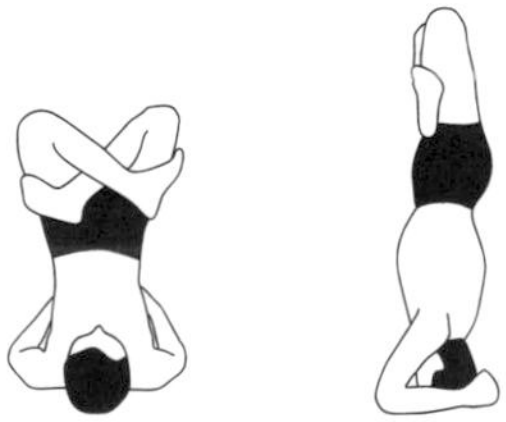

in Sarvāṅgāsana *in Śīrṣāsana*

2:27 Ūrdhva-Prasārita-Ekapādāsana
Ūrdhva - prasārita eka - pāda - āsana
Upward - spread one - leg - posture
ऊर्ध्व - प्रसारित एक - पाद - आसन
ऊर्ध्वप्रसारित एकपादासन

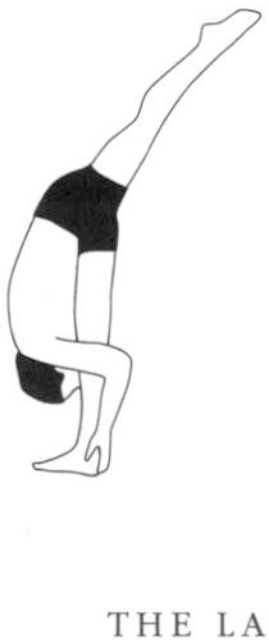

2:53 Uṣṭrāsana

Uṣṭra - āsana

Camel - posture

उष्ट्र - आसन

उष्ट्रासन

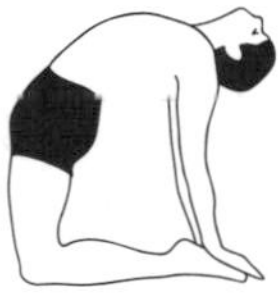

3:05 Utkaṭāsana

Utkaṭa - āsana

Fierce - posture

उत्कट - आसन

उत्कटासन

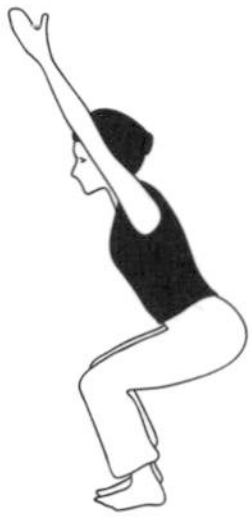

3:17 Uttānapādāsana

Uttāna - pāda - āsana

Stretched out - leg - posture

उत्तान - पाद - आसन

उत्तानपादासन

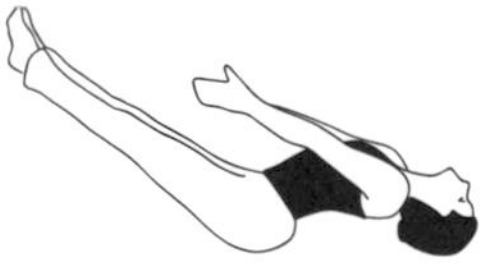

3:34 Uttāna-Padma-Mayūrāsana

Uttāna - padma - mayūra - āsana

Stretched out - lotus - peacock - posture

उत्तान - पद्म - मयूर - आसन

उत्तानपद्ममयूरासन

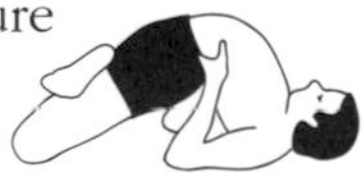

3:56 Uttānāsana

Uttāna - āsana

Stretched out - posture

उत्तान - आसन

उत्तानासन

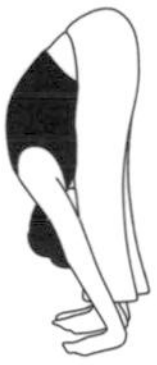

U (continued)

4:11 Utthita-Hasta-Pādāṅguṣṭhāsana

Utthita - hasta - pādāṅguṣṭha - āsana

Extended - hand - big toe - posture

उत्थित - हस्त - पादाङ्गुष्ठ - आसन

उत्थितहस्तपादाङ्गुष्ठासन

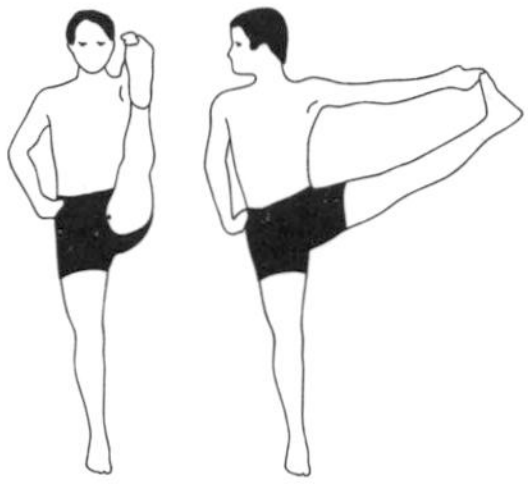

4:34 Utthita-Pārśvakoṇāsana

Utthita - pārśva - koṇa - āsana

Extended - side - angle - posture

उत्थित - पार्श्व - कोण - आसन

उत्थितपार्श्वकोणासन

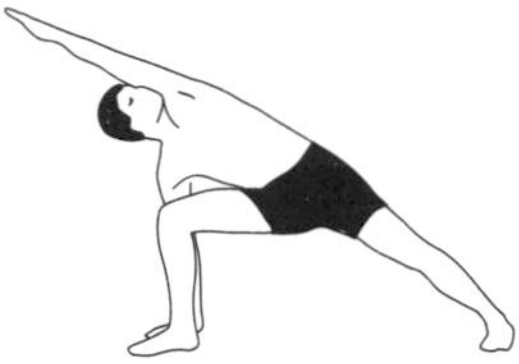

4:55 Utthita-Trikoṇāsana

Utthita - trikoṇa - āsana

Extended - triangle - posture

उत्थित - त्रिकोण - आसन

उत्थितत्रिकोणासन

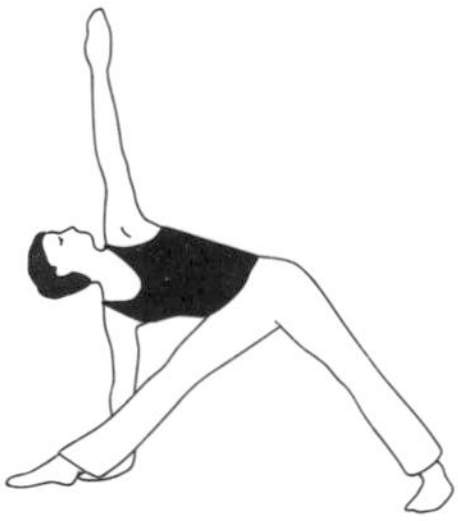

V

DISC 2, TRACK 26
Find individual postures with the time points provided.

:03 Vajrāsana
Vajra - āsana
Thunderbolt - posture
वज्र - आसन
वज्रासन

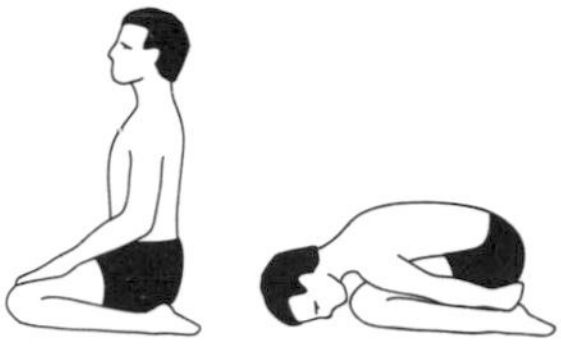

:13 Vāmadevāsana
Vāmadeva - āsana
(Name of sage) - posture
वामदेव - आसन
वामदेवासन

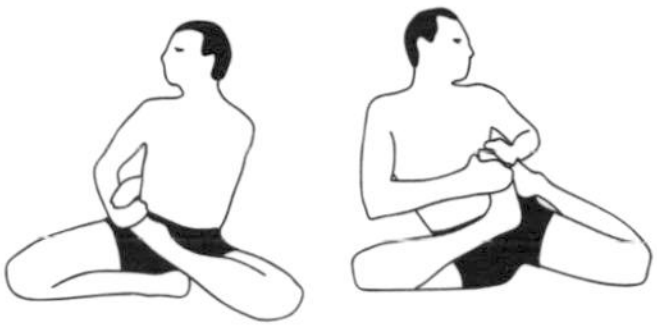

:24 Vasiṣṭhāsana
Vasiṣṭha - āsana
(Name of sage) - posture
वसिष्ठ - आसन
वसिष्ठासन

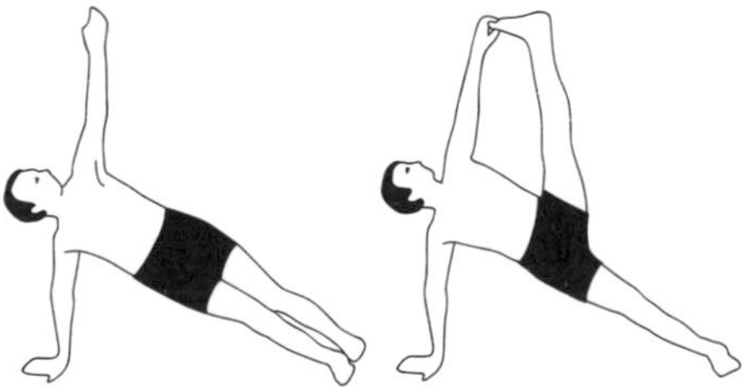

:36 Vātāyanāsana
Vātāyana - āsana
Horse - posture
वातायन - आसन
वातायनासन

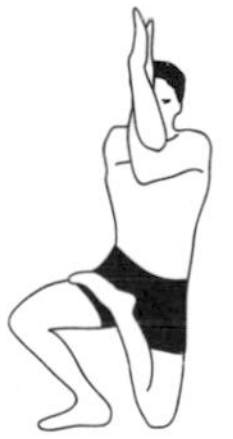

V (continued)

:49 Viparīta-Karaṇī
Viparīta - karaṇī
Inverted - doing
विपरीत - करणी
विपरीतकरणी

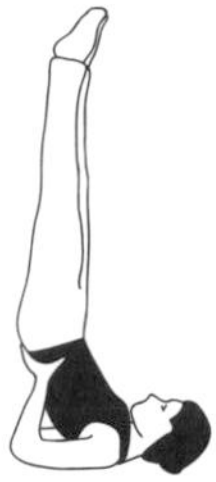

1:06 Viparīta-Śalabhāsana
Viparīta - śalabha - āsana
Inverted - locust - posture
विपरीत - शलभ - आसन
विपरीतशलभासन

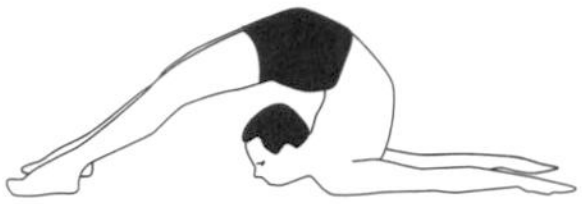

1:23 Vīrabhadrāsana
Vīrabhadra - āsana
Warrior - posture
वीरभद्र् - आसन
वीरभद्रासन

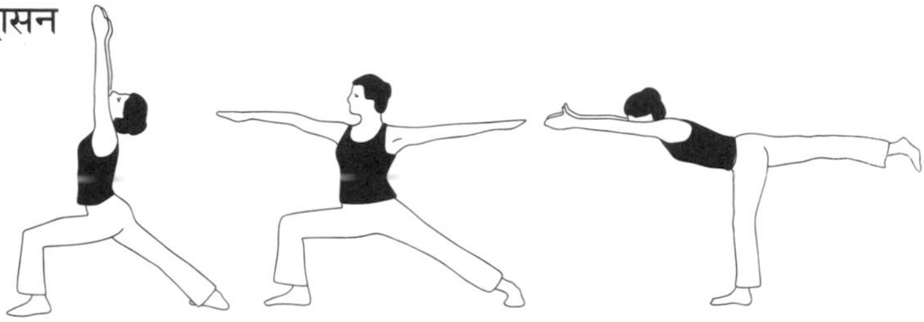

1 *2* *3*

1:36 Virañcyāsana
Virañci - āsana
(Name of sage) - posture
विरञ्चि - आसन
विरञ्च्यासन

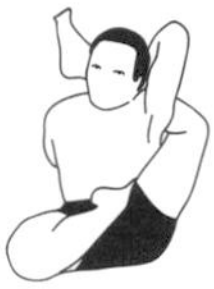

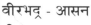

1:47 Vīrāsana
Vīra - āsana
Hero - posture
वीर - आसन
वीरासन

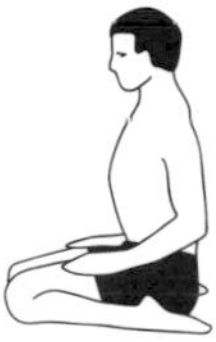

1:58 Viśvāmitrāsana
Viśvāmitra - āsana
(Name of sage) - posture
विश्वामित्र - आसन
विश्वामित्रासन

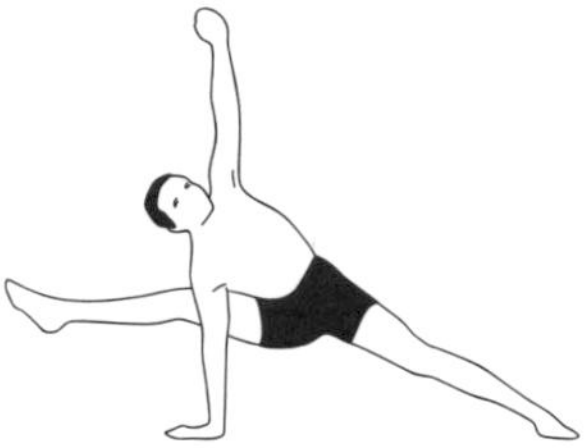

2:11 Vṛkṣāsana
Vṛkṣa - āsana
Tree - posture
वृक्ष - आसन
वृक्षासन

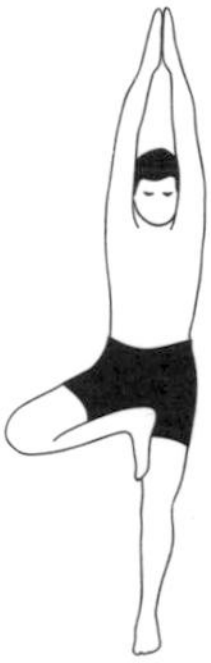

2:22 Vṛścikāsana
Vṛścika - āsana
Scorpion - posture
वृश्चिक - आसन
वृश्चिकासन

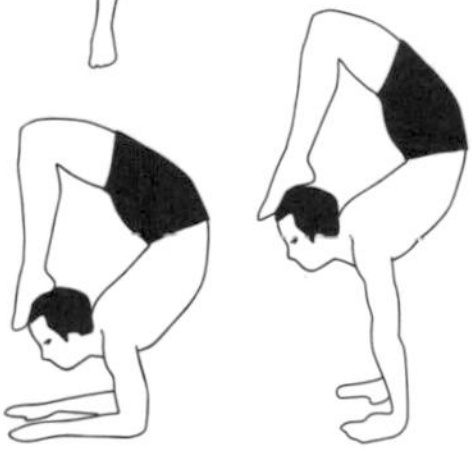

Y

DISC 2, TRACK 27
Find individual postures with the time points provided.

:03 Yoga-Daṇḍāsana
Yoga - daṇḍa - āsana
Yoga - staff - posture
योग - दण्ड - आसन
योगदण्डासन

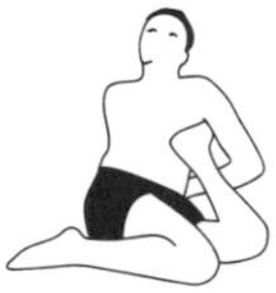

:18 Yoga-Mudrā
Yoga - mudrā
Yoga - seal
योग - मुद्रा
योगमुद्रा

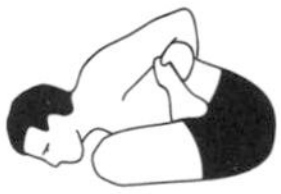

:33 Yoga-Nidrāsana
Yoga - nidrā - āsana
Yoga - sleep - posture
योग - निद्रा - आसन
योगनिद्रासन

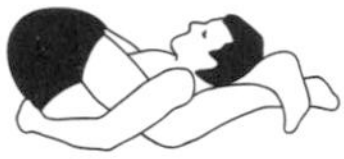

INDICES

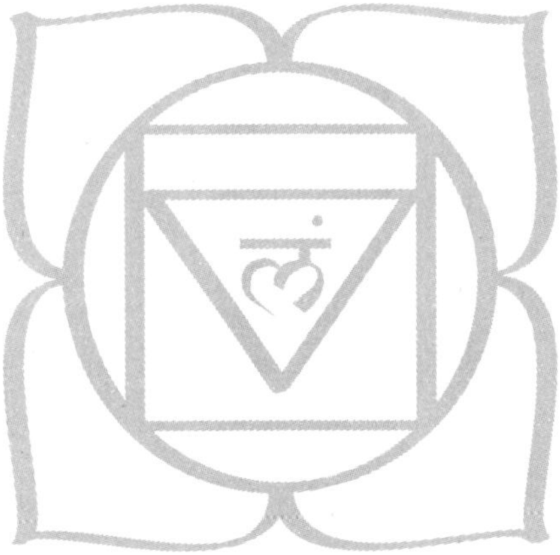

Āsana Name Synonyms

PAGE

DISC 2, TRACK 28

Adho Mukha Vīrāsana (down-faced hero)
See Bālāsana 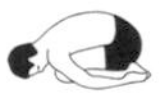 33

Añjaneyāsana (name of monkey - God)
See Hanumānāsana (same meaning) 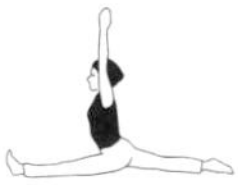 84

Brahmacaryāsana (control of vital energy)
See Upaviṣṭa - Koṇāsana (seated - angle) 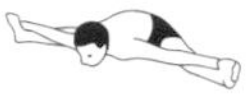 109

Bhagīrathāsana (name of sage)
See Vṛkṣāsana (tree) 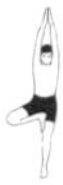 115

Hasta - Pādāsana (hand - foot)
See Pāda - Hastāsana 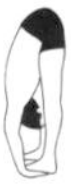 93

Jaṭhara - Parivṛtti (stomach - revolved)
See Jaṭhara - Parivartānāsana (same meaning) 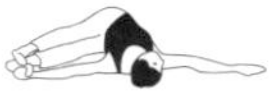 85

Kākāsana (crow)
See Bakāsana (crane) 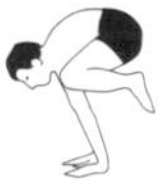 73

Kāñcyāsana (girdle)
See Mālāsana (garland) 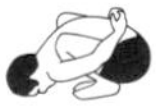 90

Maṇḍukāsana (frog)
See Bhekāsana (same meaning) 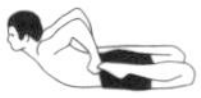 73

Matsyendrāsana (fish)
See Paripūrṇa - Matsyendrāsana (full - fish) 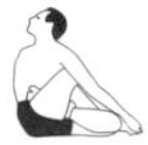 94

Mṛtāsana (dead)
See Śavāsana (corpse) 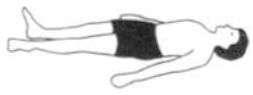 102

PAGE

Nāvāsana (boat)
See Paripūrṇa - Nāvāsana (full - boat) 94

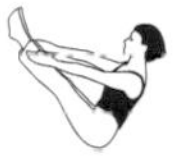

Paścimatānāsana (back - stretching)
See Paścimottānāsana (same meaning) 99

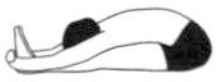

Pūrvatānāsana (front - stretching)
See Pūrvottānāsana (same meaning) 99

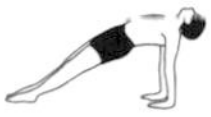

Sama - Saṃsthānam (level - position)
See Anantāsana (endless) 70

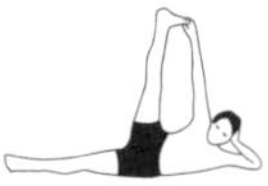

Sarvāṅgāsana (shoulderstand)
See Sālamba - Sarvāṅgāsana (supported - all - limb) 101

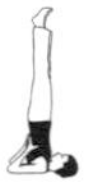

Śīrṣāsana (headstand)
See Sālamba - Śīrṣāsana (supported - head) 101

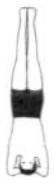

Triaṅga - Mukhaikapāda (three - limb - face...)
See Tiryaṅ - Mukhaikapāda (oblique - face...) 107

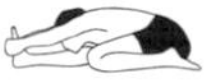

Trikoṇāsana (triangle)
See Utthita - Trikoṇāsana (extended - triangle) 112

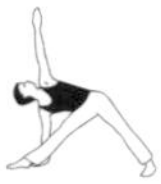

Ugrāsana (ferocious)
See Upaviṣṭa - Koṇāsana (seated - angle) 109

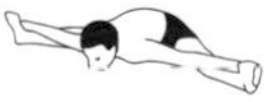

Ūrdhva - Prasārita - Pādāsana
See Supta - Daṇḍāsana 104

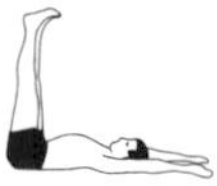

Utpluti (floating up)
See Tolāsana (balance) 108

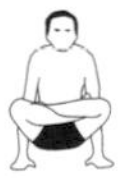

Uttāna - Mayūrāsana (stretched out - peacock)
See Setu - Bandha - Sarvāṅgāsana (bridge - lock - all - limb) 102

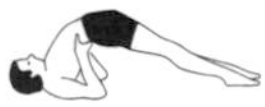

English Names

PAGE

Accomplished: Siddhāsana 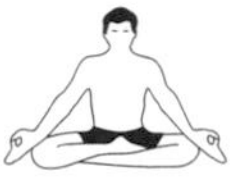 103

Airplane: Digāsana / Vīrabhadrāsana 3 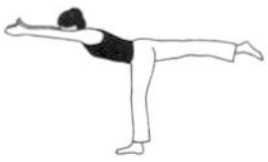 77

Alligator: Godhāpīṭham 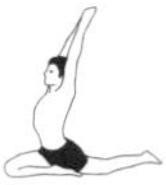 83

All - limb: Sarvāṅgāsana (Sālamba-Sarvāṅgāsana) 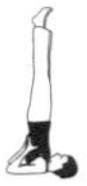 101

Arm - pressure: Bhuja-Pīḍāsana 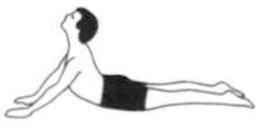 74

Auspicious: Svastikāsana 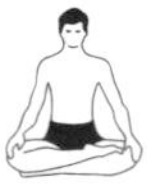 106

Back - stretched out:
Paścimottānāsana / Paścimatānāsana 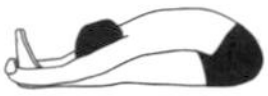 99

Ball: Piṇḍāsana (in Sarvāṅgasana) 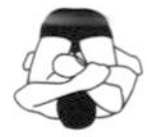 99

Beam/gate: Parighāsana 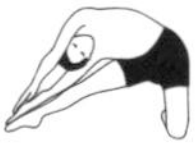 94

Bed/couch: Paryaṅkāsana 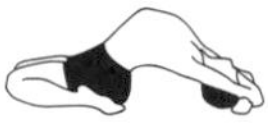 98

Bending: Ākuñcanāsana 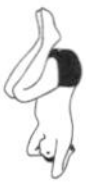 70

Big toe: Pādāṅguṣṭhāsana 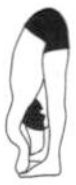 93

PAGE

Big toe - bow: Pādāṅguṣṭha - Dhanurāsana 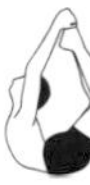 93

Bird that lives on raindrops: Kapiñjalāsana 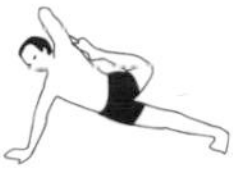 86

Boat - full: Paripūrṇa-Nāvāsana 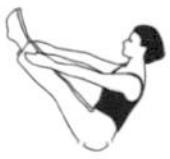 94

Boat - half: Ardha-Nāvāsana 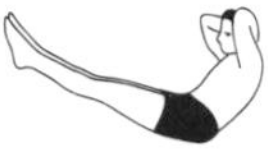 71

Both - big toe: Ubhaya-Pādāṅguṣṭhāsana 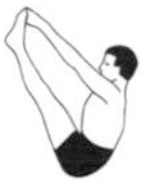 109

Bound - angle: Baddha-Koṇāsana 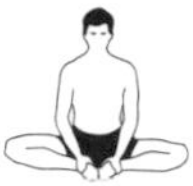 72

Bound - angle - head: Baddha-Koṇa-Śīrṣāsana 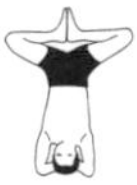 72

Bound - hand - head: Baddha-Hasta-Śīrṣāsana 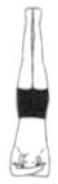 72

Bound - lotus: Baddha-Padmāsana 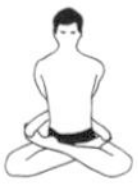 72

Bow: Dhanurāsana 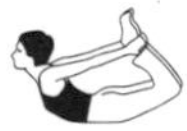 77

Bow, standing: Naṭarājāsana 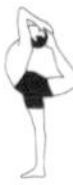 92

Bow, towards ear: Ākarṇa-Dhanurāsana 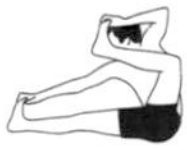 69

Bridge: Setu-Bandhāsana 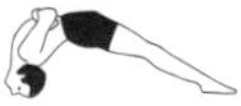 103

Bridge (one leg) in shoulderstand:
Ekapāda-Setu-Bandha-Sarvāṅgāsana 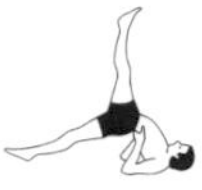 80

Bridge in shoulderstand: Setubandha-Sarvāṅgāsana 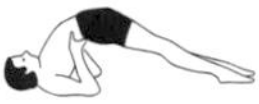 102

Buddha: Buddhāsana 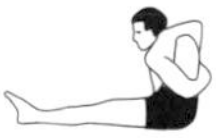 74

Butterfly: Baddha-Koṇāsana 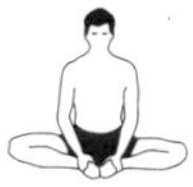 72

Cakra: Cakrāsana 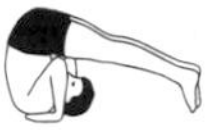 75

Camel: Uṣṭrāsana 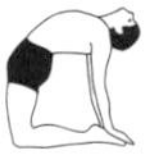 111

Cat: Cakravākāsana 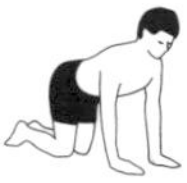 75

Child: Bālāsana 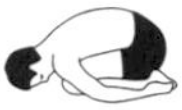 73

Circle: Maṇḍalāsana 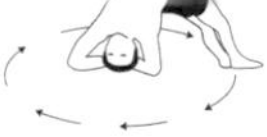 90

Cobra: Bhujaṅgāsana 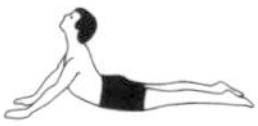 74

Comfortable: Sukhāsana 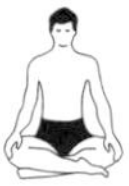 104

Corpse: Śavāsana 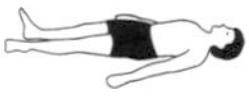 102

		PAGE
Cow - face: Go-Mukhāsana	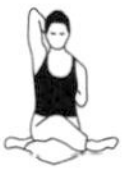	83
Cowherd: Gorakṣāsana	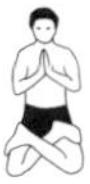	83
Crane: Bakāsana	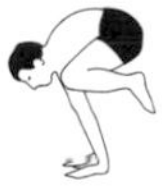	73
Crane - side: Pārśva-Bakāsana	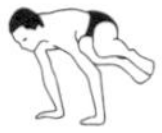	96
Crocodile: Nakrāsana (see also Makarāsana)	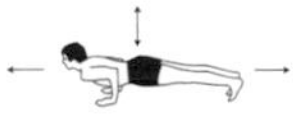	92
Cross - legged: Sukhāsana	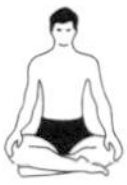	104
Crow (Kākāsana): see Bakāsana (crane)	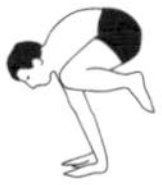	96
Dancer: Naṭarājāsana	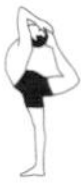	92
Dangling: Lolāsana	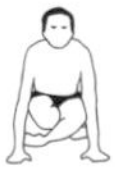	89
Dangling: Tolāsana	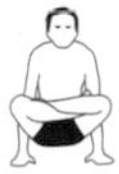	108
Dead: Śavāsana	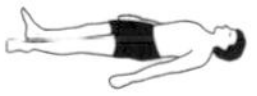	102
Direction: Digāsana / Vīrabhadrāsana 3	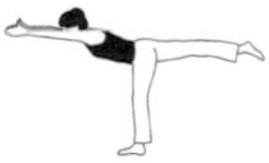	77
Dog, downward facing: Adho-Mukha-Śvānāsana	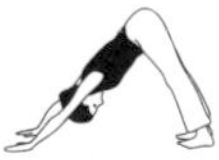	69

English Names (continued)

PAGE

Dog, upward facing: Ūrdhva-Mukha-Śvānāsana 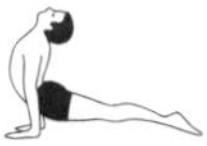 110

Downward - air: Apānāsana 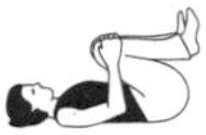 70

Downward - facing - fish: Adho-Mukha-Matsyāsana 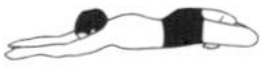 69

Downward - facing - tree: Adho-Mukha-Vṛkṣāsana 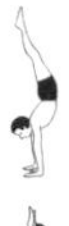 69

Eagle: Garuḍāsana 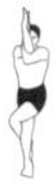 82

Ear - pressure: Karṇapīḍāsana 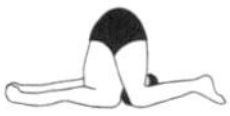 87

Easy: Sukhāsana 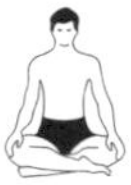 104

Endless/Viṣṇu: Anantāsana 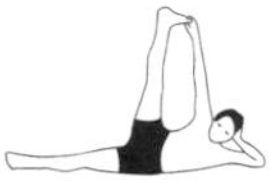 70

Equal - angle: Samakoṇāsana 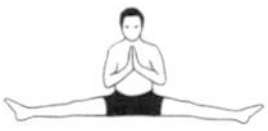 101

Equal - standing: Samasthiti 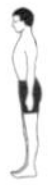 102

Extended - hand - big toe:
Utthita-Hasta-Pādāṅguṣṭhāsana 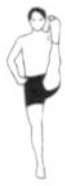 112

Extended - side - angle: Utthita-Pārśvakoṇāsana 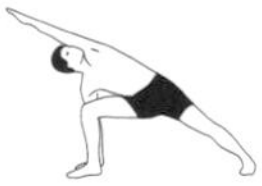 112

PAGE

Feather - peacock: Piñca-Mayūrāsana 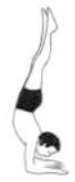 99

Firefly: Tittibhāsana 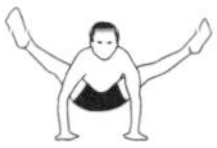 108

Fish: Matsyāsana 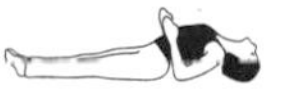 91

Fish, downward - facing: Adho-Mukha-Matsyāsana 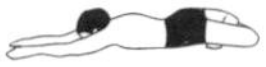 69

Fish - lord, complete: Paripūrṇa-Matsyendrāsana 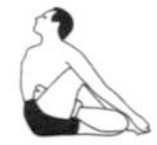 94

Fish - lord, half: Ardha-Matsyendrāsana 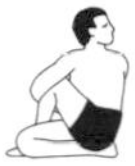 71

Foot - hand: Pāda-Hastāsana (Hastapādāsana) 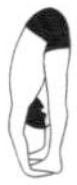 93

Formidable: Bhairavāsana  73

Forward bend: Uttānāsana 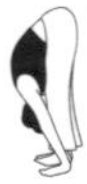 111

Forward bend, standing: Pāda-Hastāsana 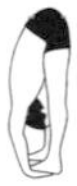 93

Frog: Bhekāsana 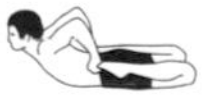 73

Front, stretched out:
Pūrvottānāsana (Pūrvatānāsana) 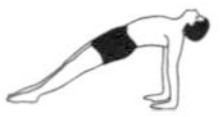 99

English Names (continued)

PAGE

Full - boat: Paripūrṇa-Nāvāsana 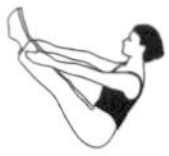 94

Garland/necklace: Mālāsana 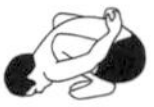 90

Gate/beam: Parighāsana 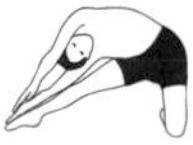 94

Half - boat: Ardha-Nāvāsana 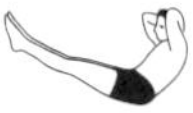 71

Half - bound - lotus, standing:
Ardha-Baddha-Padmottānāsana 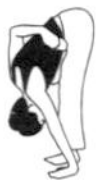 70

Half - bound - lotus, sitting:
Ardha-Baddha-Padma-Paścimottānāsana 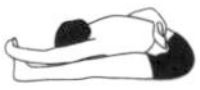 70

Half - fish - lord: Ardha-Matsyendrāsana 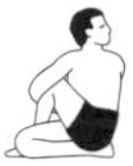 71

Half - locust: Ardha-Śalabhāsana 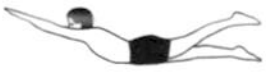 71

Half - moon: Ardha-Candrāsana 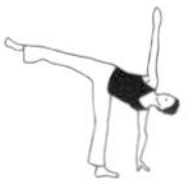 71

Handstand: Adho-Mukha-Vṛkṣāsana 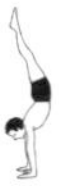 69

Head - foot: Śīrṣa-Pādāsana 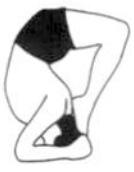 103

Headstand, bound hands: Baddha-Hasta-Śīrṣāsana 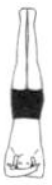 72

PAGE

Headstand, freed hands: Mukta-Hasta-Śīrṣāsana 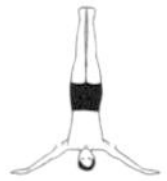 91

Headstand, one leg: Ekapāda-Śīrṣāsana 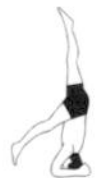 80

Headstand, revolved - one leg: Parivṛttaikapāda-Śīrṣāsana 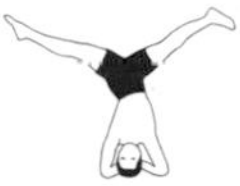 95

Headstand, side: Pārśva-Śīrṣāsana 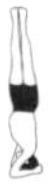 97

Headstand, side one leg: Pārśvaikapāda-Śīrṣāsana 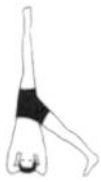 98

Headstand, two legs: Dvipāda-Śīrṣāsana 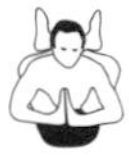 78

Headstand, supported: Sālamba-Śīrṣāsana 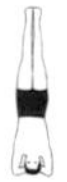 101

Hero: Vīrāsana 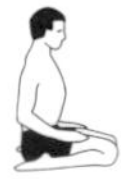 115

Heron: Krauñcāsana 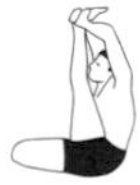 87

Himalayan goose: Kāraṇḍavāsana 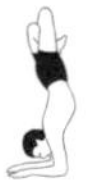 87

Horse: Vātāyanāsana 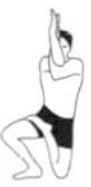 113

Inverted-doing: Viparīta-Karaṇī 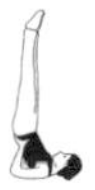 114

English Names (continued)

PAGE

Inverted - locust: Viparīta-Śalabhāsana 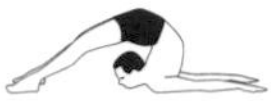 114

King - pigeon: Rāja-Kapotāsana 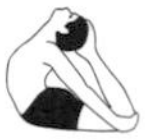 100

Knee - head: Jānu-Śīrṣāsana 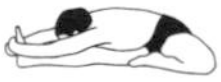 85

Knot: Kandāsana 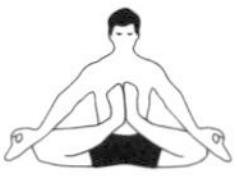 86

Light (weight) - thunderbolt: Laghu-Vajrāsana 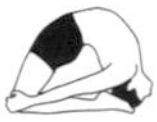 89

Lion: Siṃhāsana 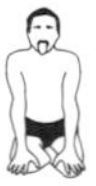 103

Lizard (iguana): Godhāpīṭham 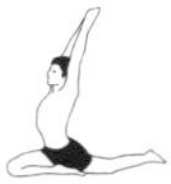 83

Locust: Śalabhāsana 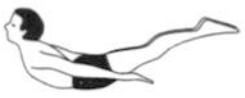 101

Lotus - peacock: Padma-Mayūrāsana 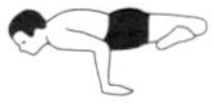 93

Lotus, full: Padmāsana 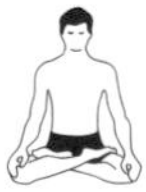 94

Mighty: Utkaṭāsana 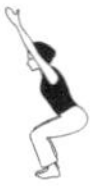 111

Moon, half: Ardha-Candrāsana 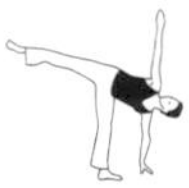 71

Mountain: Tāḍāsana 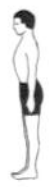 107

PAGE

Mountain: seated: Parvatāsana 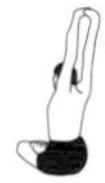 98

Mudra, great: Mahāmudrā 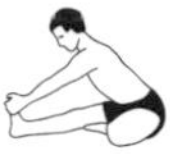 90

Mudra, six - faced: Ṣanmukhī-Mudrā 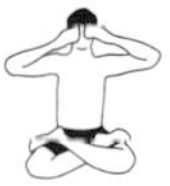 102

Mudra, yoga: Yoga-Mudrā 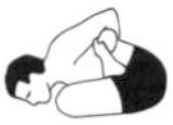 116

Noose: Pāśāsana 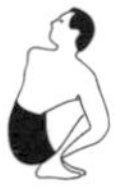 98

One - leg - (name of sage): Ekapāda-Gālavāsana 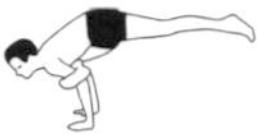 79

One - leg - (name of sage) Ekapāda-Kauṇḍinyāsana 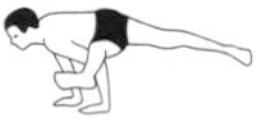 79

One - leg - crane: Ekapāda-Bakāsana 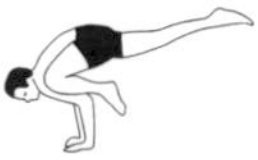 79

One - leg - inverted - staff: Ekapāda-Viparīta-Daṇḍāsana 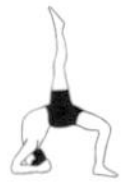 81

One - leg - king - pigeon: Ekapāda-Rāja-Kapotāsana 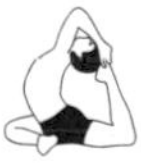 80

One - leg - upward - bow: Ekapāda-Ūrdhva-Dhanurāsana 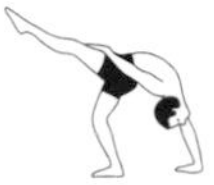 80

English Names (continued)

		PAGE
One - hand - arm: Ekahasta-Bhujāsana	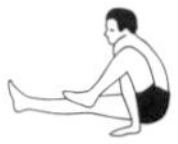	79
Partridge: Cakorāsana	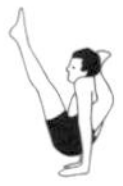	75
Peacock: Mayūrāsana	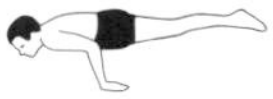	91
Peacock, extended - lotus: Uttāna-Padma-Mayūrāsana	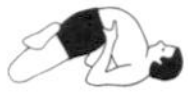	111
Peacock, lotus: Padma-Mayūrāsana	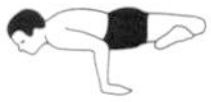	93
Peacock - feather: Pīñca-Mayūrāsana	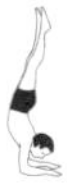	99
Pigeon: Kapotāsana	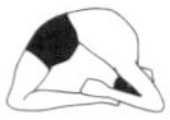	87
Plank (top of push-up): Same as Caturaṅga-Daṇḍāsana but arms are straight	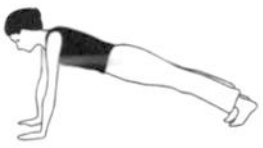	76
Plow: Halāsana	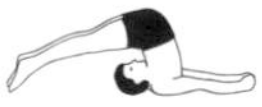	84
Plow, sideways: Pārśva-Halāsana	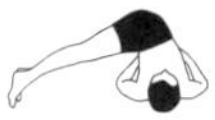	96
Reclining: See supine		
Relaxing: Śayanāsana	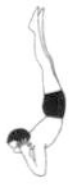	102

PAGE

Revolved - back - stretched out:
Parivṛtta-Paścimottānāsana 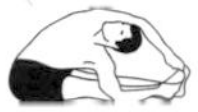 95

Revolved - half - moon:
Parivṛtta-Ardha-Candrāsana 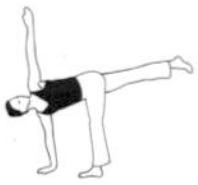 94

Revolved - knee - head: Parivṛtta-Jānu-Śīrṣāsana 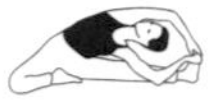 95

Revolved - side - angle: Parivṛtta-Pārśvakoṇāsana 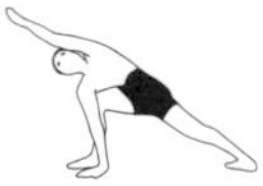 95

Revolved - triangle: Parivṛtta-Trikoṇāsana 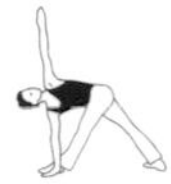 95

Rooster: Kukkuṭāsana 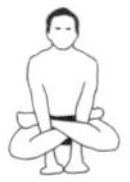 88

Rooster: upward: Ūrdhva-Kukkuṭāsana 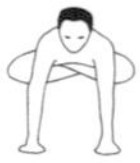 110

Root - lock: Mūlabandhāsana 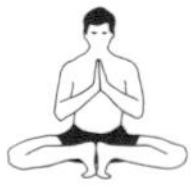 91

Ruddy goose: Cakravākāsana 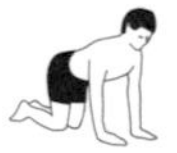 75

Scale/balance: Tolāsana 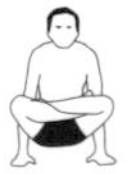 108

Scorpion: Vṛścikāsana 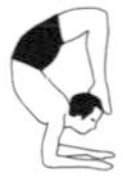 115

Seated - angle: Upaviṣṭa-Koṇāsana 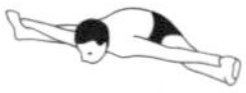 109

English Names (continued)

English Names (continued)		PAGE
Serpent/snake: Bhujaṅgāsana	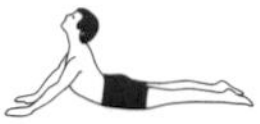	74
Shoulderstand: Sālamba-Sarvāṅgāsana	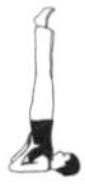	101
Shoulderstand, one leg: Ekapāda-Sarvāṅgāsana	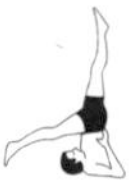	80
Shoulderstand, sideways: Pārśva-Sarvāṅgāsana	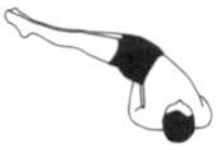	97
Shoulderstand, sideways - one - leg: Pārśvaikapāda-Sarvāṅgāsana	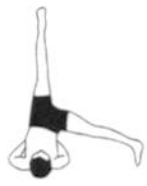	97
Shoulderstand, without support: Nirālamba-Sarvāṅgāsana	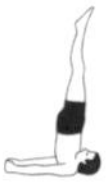	92
Side - ball: Pārśva-Piṇḍāsana (in Sarvāṅgāsana)	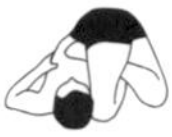	96
Side - bow: Pārśva-Dhanurāsana	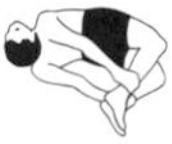	96
Side - rooster: Pārśva-Kukkuṭāsana	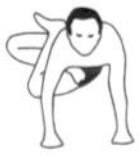	96
Side - seated - angle: Pārśva-Upaviṣṭa-Koṇāsana	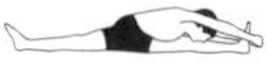	97
Side - stretched out: Pārśvottānāsana	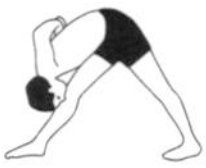	98
Side - upward - lotus: Pārśva-Ūrdhva-Padmāsana	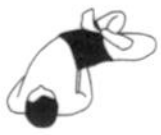	97

PAGE

Side of face - formidable: Gaṇḍa-Bheruṇḍāsana 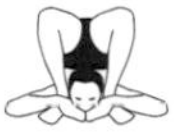 82

Six - faced seal: Ṣanmukhī-Mudrā 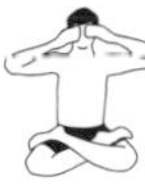 102

Split, front: Hanumānāsana 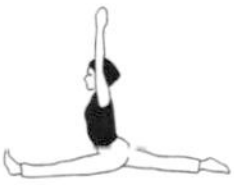 84

Split, side: Samakoṇāsana 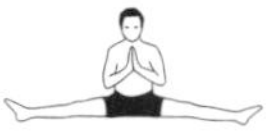 101

Split, standing: Ūrdhva-Prasārita-
Ekapādāsana / Trivikramāsana 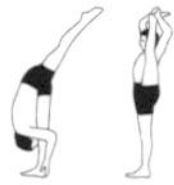 110, 108

Split, supine: Supta-Trivikramāsana  105

Spread - leg - stretched out:
Prasārita-Pādottānāsana 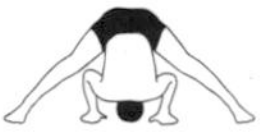 99

Squat: Mālāsana 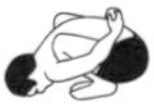 90

Staff: Daṇḍāsana 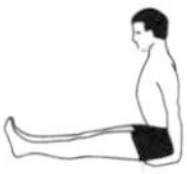 77

Staff, four - limb: Caturaṅga-Daṇḍāsana 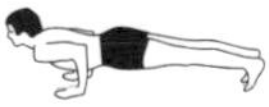 76

Staff, supine: Supta-Daṇḍāsana 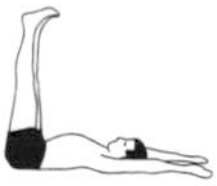 104

Staff, upward: Ūrdhva-Daṇḍāsana 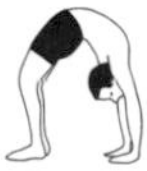 109

Stomach - revolving: Jaṭhara-Parivartanāsana 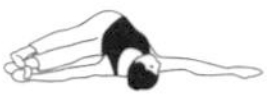 85

Stretched out - leg: Uttānapādāsana 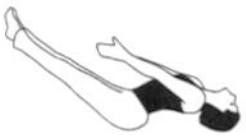 111

Sun salutation: Sūrya-Namaskāra
(for example, see Aṣṭāṅga section) 106

Supine - angle: Supta-Koṇāsana 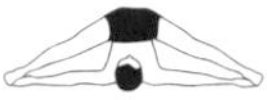 104

Supine - bound - angle: Supta-Baddha-Koṇāsana 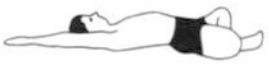 104

Supine - big toe: Supta-Pādāṅguṣṭhāsana 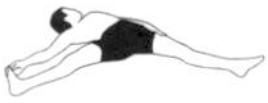 105

Supine - frog: Supta-Bhekāsana 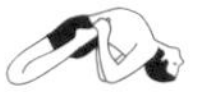 104

Supine - hero: Supta-Vīrāsana  106

Supine - staff: Supta-Daṇḍāsana 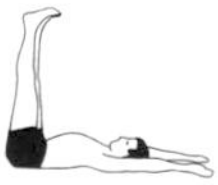 104

Supine - three - stride: Supta-Trivikramāsana 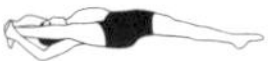 105

Supine - tortoise: Supta-Kūrmāsana 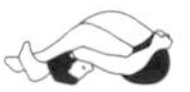 105

Supine - upwards - foot - thunderbolt:
Supta-Ūrdhva-Pāda-Vajrāsana 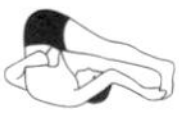 105

PAGE

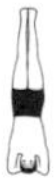
Supported headstand: Sālamba-Śīrṣāsana 101

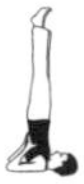
Supported shoulderstand: Sālamba-Sarvāṅgāsana 101

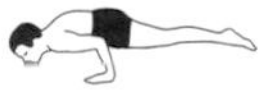
Swan: Haṃsāsana 84

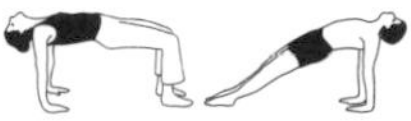
Table: Catuṣ-Pāda-Pīṭham / Pūrvottānāsana 76, 99

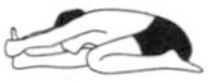
Oblique - face - one - leg - back - stretched out:
Tiryaṅ-Mukhaikapāda-Paścimottānāsana 107

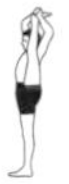
Three - stride: Trivikramāsana 108

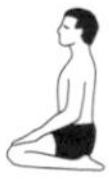
Thunderbolt: Vajrāsana 113

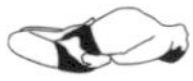
Thunderbolt, supine: Supta-Vajrāsana 105

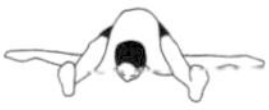
Tortoise: Kūrmāsana 88

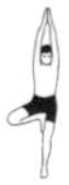
Tree: Vṛkṣāsana 115

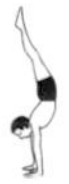
Tree, downward - facing: Adho-Mukha-Vṛkṣāsana 69

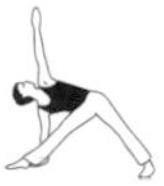
Triangle, extended: Utthita-Trikoṇāsana 112

English Names (continued) **PAGE**

Triangle, revolved: Parivṛtta-Trikoṇāsana 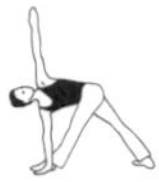 95

Two - leg: Dvipāda-Pīṭham 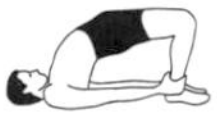 78

Two - leg - (name of sage):
Dvipāda-Kauṇḍinyāsana 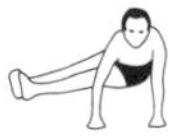 78

Two - leg - inverted - staff:
Dvipāda-Viparīta-Daṇḍāsana 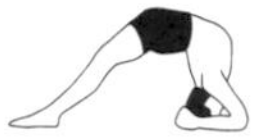 78

Two - hand - arm: Dvihasta-Bhujāsana 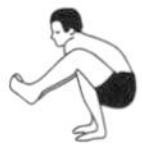 78

Upside down - face - stretched out:
Tiryaṅ-Mukhottānāsana 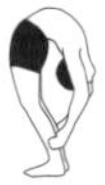 107

Upward - bow: Ūrdhva-Dhanurāsana 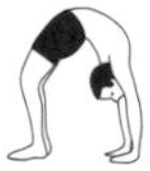 109

Upward - facing - back - stretched out:
Ūrdhva-Mukha-Paścimottānāsana 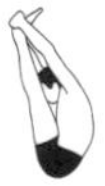 110

Upward - facing - dog:
Ūrdhva-Mukha-Śvānāsana 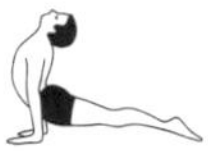 110

Upward - lotus: Ūrdhva-Padmāsana 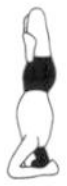 110

PAGE

Upwards - spread - one - leg:
Ūrdhva-Prasārita-Ekapādāsana 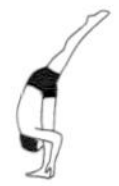 110

Warrior: Vīrabhadrāsana 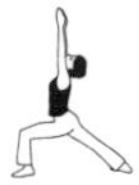 114

Wheel: Cakrāsana 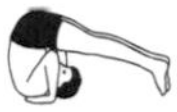 75

Wheel - lock: Cakra-Bandhāsana 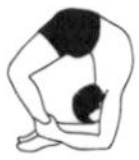 75

Womb - ball: Garbha-Piṇḍāsana 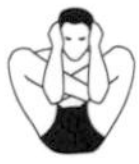 82

Yoga - seal: Yoga-Mudrā 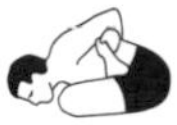 116

Yoga - sleep: Yoga-Nidrāsana 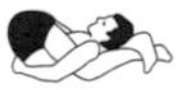 116

Yoga - staff: Yoga-Daṇḍāsana 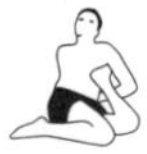 116

Sanskrit Alphabet

DISC 2, TRACK 29

14 Vowels (some have 2 forms)

अ	a	another
आ / ा	ā	father (2 beats)
इ / ि	i	pin
ई / ी	ī	need (2 beats)
उ / ु	u	flute
ऊ / ू	ū	mood (2 beats)
ऋ / ृ	ṛ	macabre
ॠ / ॄ	ṝ	trill for 2 beats
ऌ / ॢ	ḷ	table
ए / े	e	etude (2 beats)
ऐ / ै	ai	aisle (2 beats)
ओ / ो	o	yoke (2 beats)
औ / ौ	au	flautist (2 beats)

Two Special Letters

अं	aṃ	hum
अः	aḥ	out-breath

33 Consonants

क	ka	paprika
ख	kha	thick honey
ग	ga	saga
घ	gha	big honey
ङ	ṅa	ink
च	ca	chutney
छ	cha	much honey
ज	ja	Japan
झ	jha	raj honey
ञ	ña	inch
ट	ṭa	borscht again
ठ	ṭha	borscht honey
ड	ḍa	shdum
ढ	ḍha	shd hum
ण	ṇa	shnum
त	ta	pasta
थ	tha	eat honey
द	da	soda
ध	dha	good honey
न	na	banana
प	pa	paternal
फ	pha	scoop honey
ब	ba	scuba
भ	bha	rub honey
म	ma	aroma
य	ya	employable
र	ra	abra cadabra
ल	la	hula
व	va	variety
श	śa	shut
ष	ṣa	shnapps
स	sa	Lisa
ह	ha	honey